Psychiatry Essentials

A Systematic Review

Psychiatry Essentials

A Systematic Review

Alex Kolevzon, MD
Resident in Adult Psychiatry
Mount Sinai School of Medicine
New York, New York

Daphne Simeon, MD
Assistant Professor of Psychiatry
Mount Sinai School of Medicine
New York, New York

HANLEY & BELFUS, INC.

Philadelphia

Publisher: HANLEY & BELFUS, INC.
              Medical Publishers
              210 South 13th Street
              Philadelphia, PA 19107
              (215) 546-7293; 800-962-1892
              FAX (215) 790-9330
              Web site: http://www.hanleyandbelfus.com

Note to the reader: Although the information in this book has been carefully reviewed for correctness of dosage and indications, neither the author nor the publisher can accept any legal responsibility for any errors or omissions that may be made. Neither the publisher nor the author makes any warranty, expressed or implied, with respect to the material contained herein. Before prescribing any drug, the reader must review the manufacturer's current product information (package inserts) for accepted indications, absolute dosage recommendations, and other information pertinent to the safe and effective use of the product described.

Library of Congress Cataloging-in-Publication Data

Kolevzon, Alex, 1971–
    Psychiatry essentials / written by Alex Kolevzon, Daphne Simeon.
       p. ; cm.
    Includes index.
    ISBN 1-56053-483-4 (alk. paper)
    1. Psychiatry—Examinations, questions, etc. 2. Mental illness—Examinations, questions, etc. 3. Psychology, Pathological—Examinations, questions, etc. 4. Psychiatry—Handbooks, manuals, etc. 5. Mental illness—Handbooks, manuals, etc. 6. Psychology, Pathological—Handbooks, manuals, etc. I. Simeon, Daphne, 1958–II. Title.
    [DNLM: 1. Mental Disorders—Examination Questions. 2. Mental Disorders—Outlines. 3. Psychiatry—Examination Questions. 4. Psychiatry—Outlines. WM 18.2 K81p 2001]
    RC454.K595 2001
    616.89′0076—dc21   2001024712

Psychiatry Essentials   ISBN 1-56053-483-4

Last digit is the print number: 9 8 7 6 5 4 3 2 1

Dedication

To Dana, for her love and support
To Dave, for his ideas and friendship

THANK YOU

Contents

Preface

Psychiatry Essentials is a comprehensive review of clinical psychiatry presented in a unique format that will facilitate easier and more time-efficient learning. It's written from a student's perspective and answers the ongoing dilemma of which review book to rely on for clerkships and the boards. It was completed immediately after my own psychiatry clerkship, electives, and sub-internships and includes all the material I was asked on the boards and in the hospital. A unique format divides each topic into three sections to conveniently guide the reader through the material. Each section is tailored to apply to a different point during the rotation in order to maximize the efficiency of your study time. This format avoids the frustration of having to skim over all the details of any particular disorder before ever understanding any one piece of it. Rather than reading and re-reading the same pages on schizophrenia, for example, this review organizes the information in the order in which it should be learned. Each section serves as the building block for the following section and enables the reader to expand their knowledge gradually with less repetition and greater conceptual understanding.

The first two chapters of *Psychiatry Essentials,* "Approach to the Psychiatric Patient" and "The Mental Status Exam," cover topics crucial to understanding the language used to discuss patients in psychiatry. Within each subsequent chapter, the first section (The Basics) is an introductory outline that identifies and briefly describes the fundamental characteristics of all the important psychiatric disorders and treatments. This section provides the reader with a basic awareness appropriate for the first week of the rotation. The second section of each chapter (Essential Features), summarizes the essential features of all the psychiatric disorders and treatments, and the majority of study time should be dedicated to this section. Based on my own recent experience, the material in "Essential Features" will guarantee sufficient knowledge to answer most exam questions and excellent performance on the ward. "Depth and Detail" covers additional, more in-depth material that may be seen in test questions or possibly asked during the rotation. This section should be studied immediately before the exam to pick up high-yield details.

Finding a review book to rely on is always a challenge for medical students and residents. Precious time cannot be wasted on unnecessary details or tedious repetition. The introduction of *Psychiatry Essentials* signals a change in how students will study for clinical rotations and the boards. It was written because, in the already overcrowded market of review books, there are none that present the material in a format that is most useful to the student. We therefore invite you to use a review that stands apart from the rest and take a definitive step toward easier and more efficient learning.

Alex Kolevzon, MD

Approach to the Psychiatric Patient

REVIEW

The initial task of the psychiatric interview is to establish rapport with the patient. You should begin by identifying yourself and stating the purpose of the interview. The psychiatric history differs from those taken in other fields of medicine because *how* the patient relates the story is equally important to *what* they say. A psychiatrist attempts to understand personality characteristics and psychosocial dynamics as well as identifying the complaint/s. The psychiatric history does not have to follow a rigid format, but the following information should be covered in the history, and this format is adhered to in its *written* presentation.

THE PSYCHIATRIC HISTORY

I.   Identifying data
II. Chief complaint
III. History of present illness
    A. Onset
    B. Precipitating factors
IV. Past illness
    A. Psychiatric
    B. Medical
V. Personal history
    A. Prenatal and perinatal trauma
    B. Sexual abuse
    C. Physical abuse
    D. Education
    E. Alcohol or drug abuse
    F. Occupational history
    G. Marital/relationship history
    H. Social activity
    I. Religion
    J. Legal history
    K. Psychosexual history
VI. Family psychiatric history

Adapted from Kaplan HI, Sadock VA: Kaplan and Sadock's Synopsis of Psychiatry, 8th ed. Baltimore, Lippincott Williams & Wilkins, 1997.

Identifying Data
- Include the patient's name, age, sex, marital status, occupation, and current living situation.
- Language, religion, and ethnic background are sometimes also relevant details.
- Identifying data should include the setting of the interview and the source of the information.

Chief Complaint
- The chief complaint should be recorded in the patient's own words or in the words of the person who is providing the information.
- The chief complaint is typically written verbatim using quotation marks.

The Psychiatric History (continued)

History of the Present Illness (HPI)

- The HPI should chronologically describe the events leading up to the patient's presentation.
- The onset of current symptoms should be clarified and any precipitating factors described in detail.
- If the patient suffers from a chronic disorder, the course of illness to date should also be noted.

Past Illness

- Adetailed description of past psychiatric illness, hospitalizations, and treatments should be obtained.
- It should be recorded in chronological order with particular attention focused on the first episode.
- The medical history with a complete review of symptoms is also included.

Personal History

- The personal history should begin with **details of trauma,** including prenatal and perinatal trauma, sexual abuse, and physical abuse.
- **Level of education** with the last grade completed is recorded.
- An **alcohol** and **drug abuse history** with specific details of the timing and substances abused.
- **Occupational** and **marital history.**
- **Social relationships** with peers, colleagues, and siblings should be explored.
- If **religion** and **ethnicity** were not described in the identifying data, they should be here.
- A **legal history** with an assessment of **violence potential** should always be included in this section.
- Issues of sexuality, gender identity, symptoms of sexual dysfunction, and general attitudes toward sex may be asked in a **psychosexual history.**

Family Psychiatric History

- A complete review of psychiatric illness in family members, including substance abuse and suicide, should be recorded.
- Ask if family members are taking psychiatric medication or seeing a psychiatrist.

INTERVIEWING TECHNIQUES

Reflection: empathic repetition of patient's words to show understanding
Facilitation: saying yes, or uh-huh to help continue the interview
Silence: allows patient time to think or cry
Confrontation: points out something overlooked or denied
Clarification: elicits details and addresses contradictions
Transition: switches topics
Self-Revelation: limited self-disclosure to increase comfort
Reinforcement: positive feedback to encourage disclosure
Interpretation: offers insight to help awareness
Summation: summarizes information to confirm understanding
Advice: given to help patient only after they have spoken freely
Explanation: explains treatment plan, and answers questions

THE PSYCHIATRIC REPORT

- The psychiatric report should follow the outline of the psychiatric history and include a mental status exam.
- It should also include suggestions for further diagnostic work-up such as a physical exam, neurological exam, and additional interviews to gain collateral information from family members and friends.
- Positive and negative findings should *both* be summarized.

- The psychiatric report includes a proposed multiaxial diagnosis (see below).
- The end of the report should summarize the clinical impression and management recommendations.

Multiaxial Diagnosis

AXIS I clinical syndromes (including substance abuse)

AXIS II personality disorders and mental retardation

AXIS III general medical conditions

AXIS IV psychosocial stressors

AXIS V global assessment of functioning (GAF) rated from 1 to 100

Global Assessment of Functioning Scale

Code	(Note: Use intermediate codes when appropriate, e.g., 45, 68, 72.)
100 ⎪ 91	**Superior functioning in a wide range of activities, life's problems never seem to get out of hand, is sought out by others because of his or her many positive qualities. No symptoms.**
90 ⎪ 81	**Absent or minimal symptoms** (e.g., mild anxiety before an exam), **good functioning in all areas, interested and involved in a wide range of activities, socially effective, generally satisfied with life, no more than everyday problems or concerns** (e.g., an occasional argument with family members).
80 ⎪ 71	**If symptoms are present, they are transient and expectable reactions to psychosocial stressors** (e.g., difficulty concentrating after family argument); **no more than slight impairment in social, occupational, or school functioning** (e.g., temporarily falling behind in schoolwork).
70 ⎪ 61	**Some mild symptoms** (e.g., depressed mood and mild insomnia) **OR some difficulty in social, occupational, or school functioning** (e.g., occasional truancy, or theft within the household), **but generally functioning pretty well, has some meaningful interpersonal relationships.**
60 ⎪ 51	**Moderate symptoms** (e.g., flat affect and circumstantial speech, occasional panic attacks) **OR moderate difficulty in social, occupational, or school functioning** (e.g., few friends, conflicts with peers or co-workers).
50 ⎪ 41	**Serious symptoms** (e.g., suicidal ideation, severe obsessional rituals, frequent shoplifting) **OR any serious impairment in social, occupational, or school functioning** (e.g, no friends, unable to keep a job).
40 ⎪ 31	**Some impairment in reality testing or communication** (e.g., speech is at times illogical, obscure, or irrelevant) **OR major impairment in several areas, such as work or school, family relations, judgment, thinking, or mood** (e.g., depressed man avoids friends, neglects family, and is unable to work; child frequently beats up younger children, is defiant at home, and is failing at school).
30 ⎪ 21	**Behavior is considerably influenced by delusions or hallucinations OR serious impairment in communication or judgment** (e.g., sometimes incoherent, acts grossly inappropriately, suicidal preoccupation) **OR inability to function in almost all areas** (e.g., stays in bed all day; no job, home, or friends).
20 ⎪ 11	**Some danger of hurting self or others** (e.g., suicide attempts without clear expectation of death; frequently violent; manic excitement) **OR occasionally fails to maintain minimal personal hygiene** (e.g., smears feces) **OR gross impairment in communication** (e.g., largely incoherent or mute).
10 ⎪ 1	**Persistent danger of severely hurting self or others** (e.g., recurrent violence) **OR persistent inability to maintain minimal personal hygiene OR serious suicidal act with clear expectation of death.**
0	Inadequate information.

Mental Status Examination

REVIEW

The Mental Status Exam (MSE) is used to summarize the examiner's impression of the patient. It is relevant only to the time of the interview and should be used as a baseline. It is important to note that a patient's mental status may change with each examination. A thorough MSE relies on careful observation and good interviewing techniques. In formulating an impression or discussing a patient interview, always begin by summarizing the MSE.

MENTAL STATUS EXAMINATION

   I.   General Description
   II. Speech
   III. Mood and Affect
   IV. Thought Disturbance
   V.   Perceptual Disturbance
   VI. Sensorium and Cognition
   VII. Impulse Control
   VIII. Judgement and Insight
   IX. Reliability

General Description
- Describe the patient's appearance, behavior, and overall attitude toward the examiner.
- **Appearance** is described in reference to body type, posture, clothing, and grooming.
- **Behavior** refers to the presence of agitation, hyperactivity, or psychomotor retardation.
- Particular signs such as stereotyped behavior, rigidity, gait, and twitches should be noted.
- **Attitude** toward the examiner is described as cooperative, hostile, guarded, apathetic, or seductive.

Speech
- Speech is described in terms of its **quantity, rate,** and **quality.**
- Examples are talkative or sparse (quantity), rapid or slow (rate), pressured or whispered (quality).
- Record whether or not the patient's speech is spontaneous or not.
- Speech impediments and unusual rhythms (dysprosody) should also be noted.

Mood and Affect
- Mood is the patient's **internal emotional state** and is typically recorded in the patient's own words.
- Mood is described by adjectives such as depressed, anxious, euphoric, and frightened.
- Mood may be **labile** where it alternates rapidly between two extremes during an examination.
- Affect is the patient's **objective appearance** according to the examiner's impression of facial and behavioral expression.
- Affect is described as euthymic (normal), constricted, blunted, or flat.
- The normal range of affect includes variation in facial expressions, tone of voice, and body movement.
- Flat affect is defined as an immobile facial expression and monotonous voice.
- Appropriateness of affect refers to congruence between subject matter and the emotional response.

Mental Status Examination (continued)

Thought Disturbance

- Thought is divided into thought process and thought content.
- **Thought process** is the patient's ability to express ideas and the form that the thought takes.
- Illogical or incomprehensible thinking and expression of ideas is thought *process* disturbance.
- The term "thought disordered" refers specifically to the patient's thought *process* (not content).
- **Thought content** is what the person is actually thinking about.
- The most important thought *content* disturbance to elicit is recurrent ideas about suicide or homicide.
- Asking a patient about suicidal ideation will *not* trigger suicidality.

Examples of Disturbance in Thought Process

Loosening of associations: ideas are unrelated

Flight of ideas: extremely rapid thinking with fast shifts in topics

Circumstantiality: irrelevant details are included in making a point

Tangentiality: a point is never made

Thought blocking (TB): silence interrupts a train of thought

Word salad: speech is incoherent and unconnected

Clang associations: word association by rhyming

Punning: word association by double meaning

Neologisms: creation of new words

Examples of Disturbance in Thought Content

Delusions: false beliefs unrelated to culture

Ideas of reference (IOR): television or radio speaks about the patient

Ideas of influence: another force controls patient's behavior

Paranoid ideation (PI) ideas of being harmed, followed, or persecuted

Obsession: a recurrent or persistent thought or impulse

Compulsion: uncontrollable impulse to perform an act

Poverty of content: thought that is vague, repetitious, or obscure

Phobia: an unfounded fear that triggers panic

Perceptual Disturbance

- Perceptual disturbances involve the sensory system and usually present as hallucinations or illusions.
- **Hallucinations** may be visual, auditory, olfactory, gustatory, or tactile.
- A hallucination is defined as a subjective perception of an object or event that does not exist in reality and is *not* triggered by an actual stimulus.
- **Illusions** are *false* perceptions where a patient mistakes an object or event for something it is not.
- Illusions are triggered by a specific stimulus and the examiner may confuse them with hallucinations.
- A hallucination may be seeing an object that is *not* there and an illusion is misperceiving an object that *is* there.

Mental Status Examination (continued)

Sensorium and Cognition

- A Mini-Mental State Examination (MMSE) is used to assess cognitive functioning.
- The MMSE measures orientation, memory, attention, calculation, reading and writing, visuospatial relations, and language.
- The exam is scored quantitatively out of 30.
- Scores between 24 and 30 are considered normal, and scores less than 24 are indicative of dementia.
- Abstract thinking can be assessed by asking patients to explain a simple proverb such as "people who live in glass houses should not throw stones."
- Record whether answers are appropriate, too concrete, or too generalized.
- Vocabulary and knowledge are assessed by asking simple questions about current events or geography and are used to estimate overall intelligence.

Category	Examples of Instructions to Patient	Maximum Score
Orientation	**"Can you tell me the date?"**	5
	year (1), season (1), day (1), date (1), month (1)	
	"Where are you?"	5
	state (1), county (1), town (1), hospital (1), floor (1)	
Registration	**"Repeat the names of these 3 objects"**	3
	table (1), flower (1), car (1)	
Attention and Calculation	**"Subtract by 7s starting from 100"**	5
	93 (1), 86 (1), 79 (1), 72 (1), 65 (1)	
Recall	**"Recall the names of the above 3 objects"**	3
	table (1), flower (1), car (1)	
Language	**"Name the object the examiner is holding"**	2
	point to a watch (1), point to a pencil (1)	
	"Say no ifs, ands, or buts"	1
	"Take this paper in your right hand (1), **fold it in half** (1), **and put it on the floor"** (1).	3
	"Read this out loud and do what it says"	1
	show the patient a sign that says CLOSE YOUR EYES	
	"Write a sentence of your own"	1
Construction	**"Copy this design"**	1
	show the patient a pair of intersecting pentagons	

Adapted from Folstein, 1975.

Impulse Control

- Impulse control may be assessed from the patient's history and from behavior observed during the course of the interview.
- Impaired impulse control is very important to determine because it is predictive of the patient's potential danger to self or to others.

Judgement and Insight

- Judgement refers to the patient's ability to understand behavior and its consequences with respect to society.
- Ask the patient what should be done upon smelling smoke in a crowded theatre or after finding a lost child in a shopping mall.
- Insight refers to the patient's awareness and understanding of their illness.

Reliability

- Reliability refers to the patient's ability to report symptoms accurately and consistently.
- The examiner should record an impression of the patient's truthfulness and extent of disclosure.

Psychotic Disorders: The Basics

IDENTIFICATION

There are 6 psychotic disorders:

1) Brief Psychotic Disorder

2) Schizophreniform Disorder

3) Schizophrenia

4) Schizoaffective Disorder

5) Shared Psychotic Disorder

6) Delusional Disorder

CHARACTERISTICS

Psychosis is defined as a marked *impairment in reality testing.*

The classic symptoms of psychotic disorders are:
1) delusions
2) hallucinations
3) thought process disturbance (thought disorder).

A **brief psychotic disorder** is a psychosis that lasts longer than one day but less than one month.

Schizophreniform disorder is a psychosis that lasts longer than one month but less than six months.

Schizophrenia is a psychotic disorder in which the symptoms last longer than six months.

Schizoaffective disorder is diagnosed when psychotic symptoms co-exist with a prominent mood disorder. The psychotic symptoms must also be present for at least 2 weeks without the presence of the mood disorder.

Shared psychotic disorder occurs when psychotic symptoms develop in a patient in the context of a close relationship with someone who was already known to suffer from a similar psychotic syndrome.

In **delusional disorder** the main psychotic symptom is non-bizarre delusions that occur for at least one month. The most common delusions in delusional disorder are the paranoid type and the jealous type.

Psychotic Disorders: Essential Features

REVIEW

Schizophrenia is the most common psychotic disorder and the most likely cause for inpatient hospitalization. However, at the onset of psychotic symptoms the clinician must be aware of *all* the diagnostic possibilities. Schizophrenia should not be considered until symptoms are present for at least **6** months. If symptoms are present for less than 1 month, a brief psychotic disorder is the appropriate diagnosis even though schizophrenia and schizophreniform disorder still need to be ruled out. The main difference between schizophrenia, schizophreniform disorder, and brief psychotic disorder is the duration of illness. Schizoaffective disorder presents with prominent mood disturbance; delusional disorder presents with non-bizarre delusions without prominent hallucinations; and shared psychotic disorder occurs with another person. This section will review the essential features of schizophrenia and the other psychotic disorders.

ESSENTIAL FEATURES

Schizophrenia
- Schizophrenia affects 1 to 1.5 percent of the population and is equally prevalent in men and women.
- The peak age of disease onset in men is 15–25 years old, and in women is 25–35 years old.

Premorbid phase
- People with schizophrenia are generally noted to have been quiet and introverted as children.
- Patients who develop schizophrenia tend to have had few friends during adolescence.
- Odd and eccentric personality traits are often present during the premorbid phase.

Prodromal phase
- The prodromal phase may begin with somatic complaints such as pain and weakness.
- The patient's cognitive and social/occupational functioning may also begin to decline.
- Peculiar behavior with increased religiosity, bizarre ideas, and a preoccupation with philosophy or abstract ideas are common during the prodromal phase.

Active Illness
- The symptoms of schizophrenia are separated into positive and negative categories.
- Positive symptoms are hallucinations, delusions, disorganized behavior, and disorganized speech.
- Negative symptoms are **a**ffective flattening, **a**logia, **a**nhedonia, **a**pathy, and lack of **a**ttention.
- **Alogia** is defined as an inability to speak due to mental deficiency or dementia.
- **Anhedonia** is also referred to as **a**sociality, and **apathy** as **a**volition.
- Negative symptoms are sometimes remembered as the **5 As** and should not be confused with Bleuler's **4 As** which are a similar but *separate* entity (to be discussed in the following section).
- There are **5** characteristic symptoms of schizophrenia and **2** are required for diagnosis: (1) **delusions,** (2) **hallucinations,** (3) **disorganized speech,** (4) **disorganized behavior,** and (5) **negative symptoms.**
- In addition, a pattern of social and occupational deterioration is always present for at least **six months**.
- There are **5 clinical subtypes:** paranoid, disorganized, catatonic, undifferentiated, and residual.
- Patients with schizophrenia usually experience a chronic course.
- Suicide is the most common cause of death in people with schizophrenia.
- Schizophrenia is treated with antipsychotic medication that is usually required for life.

Essential Features (continued)

Brief Psychotic Disorder

- Patients with a brief psychotic disorder experience at least **1** major symptom of psychosis (delusions, hallucinations, or thought process disturbance).
- The psychotic episode lasts **less than 1 month** and then baseline premorbid functioning returns.
- Symptoms may have developed in response to a severe psychosocial stressor (reactive psychosis).
- There are three clinical subtypes: with marked stressors, without marked stressors, and postpartum.
- A postpartum brief psychotic disorder occurs within 4 weeks after delivery.
- A brief psychotic disorder is treated with antipsychotics and benzodiazepines.

Schizophreniform Disorder

- Schizophreniform disorder is clinically identical to schizophrenia.
- Its symptoms last greater than 1 month, but less than 6 months.
- Patients return to baseline premorbid functioning when the psychosis resolves.
- Prognosis is better in schizophreniform than in schizophrenia because the duration of illness is shorter.
- Schizophreniform disorder is treated with antipsychotic medication.

Schizoaffective Disorder

- Schizoaffective disorder occurs when schizophrenia and a mood disorder occur simultaneously.
- Psychotic symptoms must be present for **at least 2 weeks** in the *absence* of mood symptoms.
- Psychotic features are more likely to be **mood-incongruent** than with a mood disorder alone (depression with psychotic features).
- Mood-incongruence occurs when the content of a delusion is not consistent with the mood (e.g., a patient has command auditory hallucinations to kill him/herself despite delusions of grandeur).
- There are two clinical subtypes: bipolar type and depressive type.
- Patients generally do *not* experience the deteriorating course that is common to schizophrenia.
- The prognosis is better than in schizophrenia but worse than for mood disorders.
- Schizoaffective disorder is treated with antipsychotic medication and mood stabilizers.

Delusional Disorder

- Delusional disorder is extremely rare and the mean age of onset is approximately 40 years old.
- It is sometimes associated with recent immigration.
- Delusional disorder is characterized by delusions that are **non-bizarre** in nature.
- Non-bizarre means that the delusion is realistically possible, such as "being followed by the police."
- A patient with schizophrenia is more likely to have bizarre delusions, such as "being followed by an alien."
- Delusions in general are categorized as grandiose, paranoid, erotic, jealous, somatic, or mixed.
- Patients with delusional disorder do *not* have negative symptoms or any other positive symptoms.
- Apart from the specific impact of the delusion/s, functioning is *not* otherwise impaired.
- Delusional disorder is often resistant to antipsychotics, and psychotherapy may play a greater role.

Shared Psychotic Disorder

- Shared psychotic disorder is diagnosed after psychotic symptoms develop in the context of a close relationship with someone who was already known to suffer from a similar psychotic syndrome.
- Most cases involve two members of the same family.
- There is usually a dominant person who suffers from schizophrenia and then imposes his/her delusional system onto a younger, more passive person with dependent personality traits.
- The patient diagnosed with shared psychotic disorder does *not* have a preexisting psychiatric disorder.
- Separation from the dominant person should result in a resolution of psychotic symptoms.

Psychotic Disorders: Depth and Detail

REVIEW

Schizophrenia, the most common psychotic disorder, is characterized by delusions, hallucinations, and thought process disturbance. This section will review schizophrenia in more detail and include a historical perspective, proposed etiologies, a differential diagnosis, and the clinical subtypes.

SCHIZOPHRENIA

History

- Emil Kraepelin (1856–1926) was the first person to describe schizophrenia, and he called it *dementia praecox* (early onset).
- Eugen Bleuler (1857–1939) first used the term schizophrenia to reflect the division between thought and behavior in these patients.
- Bleuler identified 4 specific **primary symptoms** of schizophrenia known as the **4 As: A**ffect (flat), **A**utism (withdrawn), **A**ssociations (loose), and **A**mbivalence.
- The term schizophrenia is often misconstrued to mean split personality.
- Split personality is instead called dissociative identity disorder in the DSM-IV.

Epidemiology

- Schizophrenia affects approximately 1 percent of the population.
- It is equally prevalent in men and women.
- The peak age of disease onset in men is 15–25 years old and in women is 25–35 years old.
- People with schizophrenia are more likely to be in lower socioeconomic groups.

Etiology

- The **stress-diathesis model** suggests that schizophrenia is the result of a stressful environmental influence on a biological vulnerability.
- The **dopamine hypothesis** of schizophrenia states that positive symptoms result from increased dopaminergic activity.
- **Brain imaging techniques** have revealed some of the neuropathology of schizophrenia.
- The relevance of brain imaging results is unclear but it is important to be familiar with the following findings: **lateral and third ventricle enlargement on CT, hippocampal-amygdala complex reduction on MRI,** and **decreased executive functioning (prefrontal cortex) with the Wisconsin Card Sorting Test on PET.**
- A **genetic basis** for schizophrenia is widely accepted and many chromosomal markers have been implicated (heterogeneity).
- Monozygotic twins have the highest concordance rate of approximately 50 percent.
- The child of one parent with schizophrenia has a 12 percent chance of developing the disease.
- The child of two parents with schizophrenia has a 40 percent chance of developing the disease.

Schizophrenia (continued)

Diagnostic criteria for Schizophrenia

A. *Characteristic symptoms:*   Two (or more) of the following, each present for a significant portion of time during a 1-month period (or less if successfully treated):
   1. delusions
   2. hallucinations
   3. disorganized speech (e.g., frequent derailment or incoherence)
   4. grossly disorganized or catatonic behavior
   5. negative symptoms, i.e., affective flattening, alogia, or avolition
   Note: Only one Criterion A symptom is required if delusions are bizarre or hallucinations consist of a voice keeping up a running commentary on the person's behavior or thoughts, or two or more voices conversing with each other.
B. *Social/occupational dysfunction:*   For a significant portion of the time since the onset of the disturbance, one or more major areas of functioning such as work, interpersonal relations, or self-care are markedly below the level achieved prior to the onset (or when the onset is in childhood or adolescence, failure to achieve expected level of interpersonal, academic, or occupational achievement).
C. *Duration:*   Continuous signs of the disturbance persist for at least 6 months. This 6-month period must include at least 1 month of symptoms (or less if successfully treated) that meet Criterion A (i.e., active-phase symptoms) and may include periods of prodromal or residual symptoms. During these prodromal or residual periods, the signs of the disturbance may be manifested by only negative symptoms or two or more symptoms listed in Criterion A present in an attenuated form (e.g., odd beliefs, unusual perceptual experiences).
D. *Schizoaffective and Mood Disorder exclusion:*   Schizoaffective Disorder and Mood Disorder With Psychotic Features have been ruled out because either (1) no Major Depressive, Manic, or Mixed Episodes have occurred concurrently with the active-phase symptoms; or (2) if mood episodes have occurred during active-phase symptoms, their total duration has been brief relative to the duration of the active and residual periods.
E. *Substance/general medical condition exclusion:*   The disturbance is not due to the direct physiological effects of a substance (e.g., a drug of abuse, a medication) or a general medical condition.
F. *Relationship to a Pervasive Developmental Disorder:*   If there is a history of Autistic Disorder or another Pervasive Developmental Disorder, the additional diagnosis of Schizophrenia is made only if prominent delusions or hallucinations are also present for at least a month (or less if successfully treated).

From American Psychiatric Association: Diagnostic and Statistical Manual of Mental Disorders, 4th ed. Text Revision. Washington, DC, American Psychiatric Association, 2000, with permission.

Course and Prognosis
- Schizophrenia is a chronic disease that is usually lifelong.
- Cognitive functioning generally declines as the disease progresses.
- A"rule of thirds" is said to apply to prognosis: 1/3 of patients experience a deteriorating course, 1/3 have stable impairment, and 1/3 are able to function at a relatively high level.
- **Good prognostic factors** include acute or late onset; obvious precipitating factors; good premorbid functioning; and positive symptoms.
- **Poor prognostic factors** include insidious or young onset; no precipitating factors; poor premorbid functioning; and negative symptoms.
- **Suicide** is the main cause of mortality in patients with schizophrenia.
- Approximately one third of patients *attempt* suicide and 10 to 15 percent succeed.

Schizophrenia (continued)

Treatment

- Antipsychotic medication is the treatment of choice for schizophrenia.
- Mood stabilizers and benzodiazepines may be useful as adjunctive treatment.
- Behavior therapy and social skills training may improve social functioning.
- Other therapeutic options include day programs, vocational training, and residential housing.

DIFFERENTIAL DIAGNOSIS

Medical

Substance-induced (amphetamines, hallucinogens, alcohol, cocaine, PCP, and barbiturate withdrawal)

AIDS

B_{12}-deficiency

Carbon monoxide poisoning

Heavy metal poisoning

Pellagra

Wernicke-Korsakoff syndrome

Systemic lupus erythematosus

Wilson's disease

Neurological

Epilepsy (especially temporal lobe epilepsy)

Neoplasm

Cerebrovascular Disease

Trauma (especially frontal lobe or limbic)

Herpes encephalitis

Creutzfeldt-Jakob disease

Neurosyphilis

Normal pressure hydrocephalus

Psychiatric

All psychotic disorders

Major depression with psychotic features

Bipolar I disorder, manic phase

Autistic disorder

Factitious disorder

Malingering

Obsessive-compulsive disorder

Schizotypal, schizoid, borderline, and paranoid personality disorders

CLINICAL SUBTYPES

There are 5 clinical subtypes: (1) paranoid, (2) disorganized, (3) catatonic, (4) undifferentiated, and (5) residual.

Diagnostic criteria for Paranoid Type

A type of Schizophrenia in which the following criteria are met:

A. Preoccupation with one or more delusions or frequent auditory hallucinations.

B. None of the following is prominent: disorganized speech, disorganized or catatonic behavior, or flat or inappropriate affect.

Diagnostic criteria for Disorganized Type

A type of Schizophrenia in which the following criteria are met:
A. All of the following are prominent:
   1. disorganized speech
   2. disorganized behavior
   3. flat or inappropriate affect
B. The criteria are not met for Catatonic Type.

Diagnostic criteria for Catatonic Type

A type of Schizophrenia in which the clinical picture is dominated by at least two of the following:
1. motoric immobility as evidenced by catalepsy (including waxy flexibility) or stupor
2. excessive motor activity (that is apparently purposeless and not influenced by external stimuli)
3. extreme negativism (an apparently motiveless resistance to all instructions or maintenance of a rigid posture against attempts to be moved) or mutism
4. peculiarities of voluntary movement as evidenced by posturing (voluntary assumption of inappropriate or bizarre postures), stereotyped movements, prominent mannerisms, or prominent grimacing
5. echolalia or echopraxia

Diagnostic criteria for Undifferentiated Type

A type of Schizophrenia in which symptoms that meet Criterion A are present, but the criteria are not met for the Paranoid, Disorganized, or catatonic Type.

Diagnostic criteria for Residual Type

A type of Schizophrenia in which the following criteria are met:
A. Absence of prominent delusions, hallucinations, disorganized speech, and grossly disorganized or catatonic behavior.
B. There is continuing evidence of the disturbance, as indicated by the presence of negative symptoms or two or more symptoms listed in Criterion A for Schizophrenia, present in an attenuated form (e.g., odd beliefs, unusual perceptual experiences).

From American Psychiatric Association: Diagnostic and Statistical Manual of Mental Disorders, 4th ed. Text Revision. Washington, DC, American Psychiatric Association, 2000, with permission.

Mood Disorders: The Basics

IDENTIFICATION

There are 5 mood disorders:

1) Major Depressive Disorder

2) Dysthymic Disorder

3) Bipolar I Disorder

4) Bipolar II Disorder

5) Cyclothymic Disorder

CHARACTERISTICS

The symptoms of a depressive episode are:
1) depressed mood
2) disturbed sleep
3) loss of interest/pleasure
4) feelings of guilt
5) loss of energy
6) impaired concentration
7) changes in appetite
8) psychomotor changes
9) suicidal ideation

The symptoms of a manic episode are:
1) elevated *or* irritable mood
2) inflated self-esteem
3) decreased need for sleep
4) pressured speech
5) racing thoughts
6) increased distractibility
7) increased goal-directed activity
8) hedonism/hypersexuality

Major Depressive Disorder is characterized by a depressed mood *or* loss of interest or pleasure with **4** other symptoms of depression for at least 2 *weeks.*

Dysthymic Disorder is diagnosed when a depressed mood and **2** other symptoms of depression are present for at least 2 *years.* The symptoms of dysthymic disorder are similar to major depressive disorder except they are less severe and must occur over a longer duration of time (2yrs vs. 2wks).

Bipolar I Disorder is characterized by mood fluctuations between manic and major depressive episodes. Bipolar I disorder is diagnosed after a single manic episode with persistently **elevated** mood and **3** other symptoms of mania for at least *1 week.* A persistently **irritable** mood with **4** other symptoms of mania for at least 1 week also meets the diagnostic requirements for bipolar I disorder.

Bipolar II Disorder is diagnosed in the presence (or history) of a major depressive episode **and** the presence (or history) of a hypomanic episode. The main difference between mania and a hypomania is that a hypomanic episode is less severe and does *not* cause marked impairment in functioning. The difference between the 2 bipolar disorders is that bipolar II disorder *cannot* be diagnosed in the presence (or history) of a manic episode.

Cyclothymic Disorder is characterized by mood fluctuations between hypomanic and dysthymic symptoms over the course of at least *2 years.* Cyclothymic disorder is a less severe form of bipolar I disorder. It can *not* be diagnosed in the presence (or history) of a major depressive or manic episode.

Mood Disorders: Essential Features

REVIEW

The two main mood disorders are major depression and bipolar I. Major depression is unipolar and the patient experiences only major depressive episodes. Bipolar I disorder is characterized by cycling between major depressive episodes and manic episodes. Dysthymia is a milder form of major depression that occurs chronically over at least 2 years. Cyclothymia is a milder form of bipolar I with hypomanic (not manic) and dysthymic symptoms that also occur chronically over at least 2 years. Bipolar II is thought to be its own entity and is characterized by fluctuations between hypomanic and major depressive episodes. The proposed etiology of the mood disorders is a combination of genetic predisposition, neurotransmitter dysregulation, and psychosocial factors. Mood disorders are treated with psychotherapy and antidepressant or mood stabilizing medication. This section will review the essential features of the mood disorders.

ESSENTIAL FEATURES

Major Depressive Disorder

- There are **9** major symptoms of MDD and **5** (including depressed mood) are required for diagnosis: (1) depressed mood, (2) sleep disturbance, (3) loss of interest, (4) feelings of guilt, (5) low energy, (6) impaired concentration, (7) changes in appetite, (8) psychomotor changes, and (9) suicidal ideation.
- **Depressed mood** and a **loss of interest or pleasure** (anhedonia) in activities are the hallmarks.
- Patients frequently experience a loss of enjoyment in sexual activity and decreased libido.
- **Sleep problems** are extremely common in MDD and include hypersomnia and insomnia (difficulty falling asleep, difficulty staying asleep, and/or early morning awakening).
- **Guilt** is typically manifested by feelings of worthlessness or regrets about the past.
- **Energy** is almost always decreased or absent and the patient may have difficulty getting out of bed.
- **Concentration** is often affected, and reading or watching television may be intolerable.
- **Appetite** changes are usually anorexia with accompanying weight loss.
- Hyperphagia and weight gain are characteristic of *atypical* depression (a mood disorder specifier).
- **Psychomotor agitation** or **psychomotor retardation** is often present.
- **Suicidal ideation** occurs in approximately two-thirds of patients with MDD.
- An increased risk of suicide is associated with feelings of **hopelessness.**
- An irritable mood is more likely to be present in children who suffer from MDD.
- Psychotic symptoms such as delusions and hallucinations may occur in MDD (major depression with psychotic features), particularly in older populations.
- Symptoms of depression are often worse in the morning and improve over the course of the day (diurnal variation).
- MDD has a variable course with patients suffering from symptoms in *discrete* episodes.
- Although less than half of patients seek treatment, the vast majority can be treated successfully.
- MDD is treated with a combination of psychotherapy and antidepressant medication.
- Electroconvulsive therapy (ECT) may be considered in cases of refractory or psychotic depression.

Essential Features (continued)

Dysthymic Disorder

- There are 7 symptoms of dysthymic disorder and 3 (including depressed mood) are required for diagnosis: (1) depressed mood, (2) appetite changes, (3) sleep changes, (4) loss of energy, (5) low self-esteem, (6) poor concentration, and (7) feelings of hopelessness.
- Dysthymic disorder with a superimposed major depressive episode is an entity known as "double depression."
- Dysthymic disorder is a chronic illness *without* discrete symptomatic periods (such as in MDD).
- Suicidal ideation, psychomotor agitation, and psychomotor retardation are *not* characteristic.
- It is treated with psychotherapy and antidepressant medication.

Bipolar I Disorder

- Bipolar I disorder affects 1 percent of the population and is *equally* prevalent in men and women.
- Bipolar I disorder can be diagnosed after a single manic episode, but is typically characterized by cycling between manic and major depressive episodes.
- A manic episode may have 8 symptoms and 4 (including elevated mood) are required for diagnosis: (1) elevated *or* irritable mood, (2) inflated self-esteem, (3) decreased need for sleep, (4) pressured speech, (5) racing thoughts, (6) increased distractibility, (7) increased goal-directed activity, and (8) hedonism.
- If the mood is described as irritable, then 4 *additional* symptoms of mania must be present.
- The **elevated mood** lasts at least one week unless hospitalization is required, and then any duration is sufficient to diagnose a manic episode.
- **Inflated self-esteem** is often apparent through *mood-congruent* delusions of grandeur with themes of exaggerated power, intelligence, and worth.
- During a manic episode patients may not **sleep** at all or claim to feel rested after only 3 hours.
- Patients become extremely talkative with rapid, **pressured speech.**
- The thought process is often disturbed with flight of ideas or they may describe **racing thoughts.**
- Manic patients have difficulty focusing on only one task at a time and they are **easily distractible.**
- They may tell you they are working on many different projects simultaneously and appear to be psychomotor agitated with **increased goal-directed activity.**
- **Hedonism** is manifested by hypersexuality or impulsive and excessive money spending.
- The majority of patients with bipolar I disorder experience a chronic course that requires long-term prophylactic treatment with mood stabilizers.
- Psychotherapy is important to help patients gain insight and recognize the need for treatment, and also to cope with stressors.

Bipolar II Disorder

- Bipolar II disorder is characterized by mood fluctuations between hypomania and *major* depression.
- Bipolar II disorder is less severe than bipolar I because hypomanic symptoms do not cause as much distress as manic symptoms and do not require hospitalization.
- It is a chronic disease that requires psychotherapy and treatment with mood stabilizers.
- Antidepressant medication is likely to induce hypomania or mania in these patients.

Essential Features (continued)

Cyclothymic Disorder

- Cyclothymic disorder is characterized by hypomanic and depressive symptoms for at least 2 years.
- Depressive symptoms are less severe than in MDD and more consistent with dysthymia.
- A manic episode has never occurred.
- Patients with cyclothymic disorder often experience periods of mixed symptoms.
- Changes of mood may be abrupt and the cycles of this disorder are usually shorter than in bipolar I.
- Irritability is a common symptom.
- Cyclothymia is a chronic disorder that requires treatment with mood stabilizers.
- Psychotherapy may help the patient develop effective coping strategies.

Mood Disorders: Depth and Detail

REVIEW

Mood disorders are among the most common psychiatric diagnoses. The clinical presentation of mood disorders occurs along a spectrum from major depression to mania. Dysthymia, euthymia (normal mood), and hypomania lie on a continuum between the poles of depression and mania. This section will review the significant details of the mood disorders as well as a differential diagnosis and the specific features that are sometimes described for diagnostic utility (mood disorder specifiers).

MAJOR DEPRESSIVE DISORDER

Epidemiology

- Prevalence estimates of major depressive disorder (MDD) vary widely but it may affect up to 10 percent of men and 20 percent of women at some point in their lifetime.
- The mean age of onset is 40 years old but MDD can also occur in children and the elderly.
- Race and socioeconomic status do not appear to be factors in the development of mood disorders.

Etiology

- There is strong evidence in support of **genetic factors** influencing the development of MDD.
- It is theorized that mood disorders may be related to **dysregulation** of the biological amines: serotonin, norepinephrine, dopamine.
- **Psychosocial factors,** such as past or present trauma (e.g., loss of a parent or spouse), increase the likelihood of developing MDD.
- **Medical illness,** such as heart disease or stroke, may increase the risk of developing MDD.

Diagnostic criteria for Major Depressive Episode

A. Five (or more) of the following symptoms have been present during the same 2-week period and represent a change from previous functioning; at least one of the symptoms is either (1) depressed mood or (2) loss of interest or pleasure.

   Note: Do not include symptoms that are clearly due to a general medical condition, or mood-incongruent delusions or hallucinations.

   (1) depressed mood most of the day, nearly every day, as indicated by either subjective report (e.g., feels sad or empty) or observation made by others (e.g., appears tearful).   **Note:** In children and adolescents, can be irritable mood.

   (2) markedly diminished interest or pleasure in all, or almost all, activities most of the day, nearly every day (as indicated by either subjective account or observation made by others)

   (3) significant weight loss when not dieting or weight gain (e.g., a change of more than 5% of body weight in a month), or decrease or increase in appetite nearly every day.   **Note:** In children, consider failure to make expected weight gains.

   (4) insomnia or hypersomnia nearly every day

   (5) psychomotor agitation or retardation nearly every day (observable by others, not merely subjective feelings of restlessness or being slowed down)

   (6) fatigue or loss of energy nearly every day

Major Depressive Disorder (continued)

(7) feelings of worthlessness or excessive or inappropriate guilt (which may be delusional) nearly every day (not merely self-reproach or guilt about being sick)

(8) diminished ability to think or concentrate, or indecisiveness, nearly every day (either by subjective account or as observed by others)

(9) recurrent thoughts of death (not just fear of dying), recurrent suicidal ideation without a specific plan, or a suicide attempt or a specific plan for committing suicide

B. The symptoms do not meet criteria for a Mixed Episode.

C. The symptoms cause clinically significant distress or impairment in social, occupational, or other important areas of functioning.

D. The symptoms are not due to the direct physiological effects of a substance (e.g., a drug of abuse, a medication) or a general medical condition (e.g., hypothyroidism).

E. The symptoms are not better accounted for by Bereavement, i.e, after the loss of a loved one, the symptoms persist for longer than 2 months or are characterized by marked functional impairment, morbid preoccupation with worthlessness, suicidal ideation, psychotic symptoms, or psychomotor retardation.

From American Psychiatric Association: Diagnostic and Statistical Manual of Mental Disorders, 4th ed., Text Revision. Washington, DC, American Psychiatric Association, 2000, with permission.

Course and Prognosis

- Major depressive disorder has a variable course with discrete symptomatic periods.
- Depressive episodes are self-remitting and will typically last between 6 and 12 months if untreated.
- Functioning usually returns to baseline after the depressive episode subsides.
- The disorder may be chronic and require lifelong prophylaxis with antidepressant medication.
- Approximately 75 percent of patients can be treated successfully.
- The major complication of MDD is suicide.
- Approximately 15 percent of patients with MDD will eventually commit suicide.

Treatment

- Less than half of patients with depression will seek treatment.
- MDD is usually treated with a combination of psychotherapy and antidepressant medication.
- There are several different classes of antidepressants used in MDD (see "antidepressants" for a full discussion).
- Major depression with psychotic features may require treatment with antipsychotic *and* antidepressant medication.
- In the treatment of MDD, antidepressants should be given for at least **6** months from the point of remission.
- If major depressive episodes recur, more long-term prophylaxis is indicated.
- ECT is used in cases of treatment-resistant depression, depression with psychotic features, or acutely suicidal patients.

DYSTHYMIC DISORDER

Epidemiology

- Dysthymic disorder affects 3 to 5 percent of the population.
- It is more common in women than in men.
- It frequently co-exists with other psychiatric conditions such as anxiety and major depression.
- Dysthymia and MDD together are an entity known as "**double depression.**"

Dysthmic Disorder (continued)

Etiology

- Dysthymia is conceptualized as a less severe form of MDD, so its etiology is considered to be similar.

Course and Prognosis

- Dysthymia is a chronic illness *without* discrete symptomatic episodes (such as in MDD).
- The severity of the disorder may wax and wane but symptoms are present for at least 2 years.
- Some patients may go on to develop major depression.

Treatment

- Dysthymic disorder is treated with a combination of psychotherapy and antidepressant medication.
- The psychotherapeutic technique with the most objective support is cognitive-behavioral therapy.
- The same classes of antidepressant medications are used for dysthymia as for MDD.

BIPOLAR I DISORDER

Epidemiology

- Bipolar I disorder affects 1 percent of the population, and is much less common than MDD.
- It is *equally* prevalent in men and women.
- The mean age of onset of bipolar I disorder is 30 years old, but it also occurs in children and adolescents.

Etiology

- Biogenic amine dysregulation, genetic factors, and psychosocial stressors all play a role in the etiology of bipolar I disorder.

Diagnostic criteria for Manic Episode

A. A distinct period of abnormally and persistently elevated, expansive, or irritable mood, lasting at least 1 week (or any duration if hospitalization is necessary).

B. During the period of mood disturbance, three (or more) of the following symptoms have persisted (four if the mood is only irritable) and have been present to a significant degree:
  (1) inflated self-esteem or grandiosity
  (2) decreased need for sleep (e.g., feels rested after only 3 hours of sleep)
  (3) more talkative than usual or pressure to keep talking
  (4) flight of ideas or subjective experience that thoughts are racing
  (5) distractibility (i.e., attention too easily drawn to unimportant or irrelevant external stimuli)
  (6) increase in goal-directed activity (either socially, at work or school, or sexually) or psychomotor agitation
  (7) excessive involvement in pleasurable activities that have a high potential for painful consequences (e.g., engaging in unrestrained buying sprees, sexual indiscretions, or foolish business investments)

C. The symptoms do not meet criteria for a Mixed Episode

D. The mood disturbance is sufficiently severe to cuase marked impairment in occupational functioning or in usual social activities or relationships with others, or to necessitate hospitalization to prevent harm to self or others, or there are psychotic features.

E. The symptoms are not due to the direct physiological effects of a substance (e.g., a drug of abuse, a medication, or other treatment) or a general medical condition (e.g., hyperthyroidism).

  Note: Manic-like episodes that are clearly caused by somatic antidepressant treatment (e.g., medication, electroconvulsive therapy, light therapy) should not count toward a diagnosis of Bipolar I Disorder.

From American Psychiatric Association: Diagnostic and Statistical Manual of Mental Disorders, 4th ed. Text Revision. Washington, DC, American Psychiatric Association, 2000, with permission.

Bipolar I Disorder (continued)

Course and Prognosis

- The onset of bipolar I disorder usually occurs with a depressive episode.
- The diagnosis *cannot* be made until a manic episode occurs.
- Almost 90 percent of patients have more than 1 episode *or* develop a chronic course.
- Prognosis depends on the number and duration of manic episodes and premorbid functioning.

Treatment

- Long-term prophylaxis is achieved with mood stabilizers.
- Antipsychotics are used to treat *acute* mania with *or* without symptoms of psychosis.
- *Acute* mania is also treated with benzodiazepines for sedation.
- The most significant obstacle to treatment in these patients is their characteristic lack of insight.
- It may take many hospitalizations before a patient recognizes the need for prophylactic treatment.

BIPOLAR II DISORDER

Epidemiology

- The lifetime prevalence of bipolar II disorder is 0.5 percent.

Etiology

- Bipolar II disorder may be a separate entity from bipolar I disorder.
- There is some evidence to suggest that bipolar II is related to borderline personality disorder.
- Biogenic amine dysregulation and psychosocial factors influence the development of the disorder.
- Genetic factors also play a role because there is a pattern of familial inheritance in bipolar II.

Course and Prognosis

- Bipolar II disorder is considered a chronic disease that requires long-term treatment

Treatment

- Psychotherapy, mood stabilizers, and antidepressant medication are all used to treat bipolar II disorder.
- Antidepressant medication must be used cautiously in these patients because they are highly susceptible to anti-depressant-induced mania.

CYCLOTHYMIC DISORDER

Epidemiology

- Cyclothymic disorder affects approximately 1 percent of the general population.
- It is more common in the psychiatric population and may co-exist with borderline personality disorder.
- Cyclothymia is equally prevalent in men and women (like bipolar I).

Etiology

- Cyclothymia is a less severe form of bipolar I disorder and its etiology is considered to be similar.

Course and Prognosis

- Cyclothymic disorder has a chronic course, and prognosis is dependent on individual coping strategies.
- Approximately one-third of patients are eventually diagnosed with bipolar I disorder.

Cyclothymic Disorder (continued)

Treatment

- Mood stabilizers are the treatment of choice for cyclothymic disorder.
- Antidepressants are likely to induce hypomania or mania in these patients.

DIFFERENTIAL DIAGNOSIS

Medical

Hypothyroidism (frequently asked differential for MDD)

HIV/AIDS

Viral infection (especially EBV)

Chronic disease (SLE, anemia, diabetes)

Cancer (especially pancreatic for MDD)

Medications (cardiac drugs, corticosteroids, antipsychotics, oral contraceptives, stimulants, and analgesics).

Neurological

Parkinson's disease

Dementia

Epilepsy

Tumors

Multiple sclerosis

Psychiatric

Substance abuse disorders

Schizoaffective disorder

Eating disorders

Somatoform disorders

Anxiety disorders

Borderline personality disorder

Bereavement

- The symptoms of bereavement may be indistinguishable from **MDD.**
- Uncomplicated bereavement usually **remits spontaneously within 6 months to 1 year.**
- The diagnosis of MDD should be considered in a bereaved person if *any* of the following are present: (1) *severe* functional impairment, (2) psychosis, (3) suicidal ideation, (4) feelings of worthlessness, or (5) psychomotor retardation.

Adjustment Disorder

- An adjustment disorder with depressed mood may appear clinically similar to **MDD** *or* **dysthymia,** but is less severe and with fewer depressive symptoms.
- An **identifiable cause** is necessary to distinguish between an adjustment disorder and a primary mood disturbance.
- Adjustment disorder can be diagnosed only in the presence of an identifiable psychosocial stressor within the **past 3 months.**
- If the stressor is removed, symptoms should resolve within **6** months.
- If a patient meets diagnostic criteria for MDD or dysthymia, it is considered MDD or dysthymia regardless of the presence of an identifiable cause.

MOOD DISORDER SPECIFIERS

There are 7 clinical *specifiers* of mood disorders: melancholic features, postpartum onset, catatonic features, atypical features, seasonal pattern, rapid cycling, and chronic specifier. These specifiers are distinct from the clinical *subtypes* used in other disorders (e.g., psychotic disorders).

Melancholic Features Specifier
- Melancholic features can apply to MDD, bipolar I, and bipolar II disorder.
- Melancholia is a more severe form of major depression.
- It is characterized by a loss of pleasure in almost all activities (anhedonia).
- Patients feel *excessively* guilty and may experience significant anorexia with weight loss.
- Early morning exacerbation of symptoms with improvement over the course of the day is especially characteristic of melancholia.

Postpartum Onset Specifier
- Postpartum onset can apply to MDD, bipolar I, bipolar II, *and* brief psychotic disorder.
- This specifier is used if the onset of the disorder occurred within **4** weeks postpartum.

Catatonic Features Specifier
- Catatonic features can apply to MDD, bipolar I, and bipolar II disorder.
- There are 5 symptoms of catatonia, and 2 are required for diagnosis: (1) motoric immobility, (2) excessive motor activity, (3) extreme negativism, (4) bizarre voluntary movement, and (5) echolalia and echopraxia.

Atypical Features Specifier
- Atypical features can apply to MDD, bipolar I, bipolar II, *and* dysthymic disorder.
- These patients tend to experience mood improvement in response to positive events.
- They are classically *hyper*somniacs who show *increased* appetite and significant weight gain.
- Leaden paralysis, a heavy feeling in the arms and legs, is often attributed to catatonic features but is actually more characteristic of an *atypical* presentation.

Seasonal Pattern Specifier
- Seasonal pattern can be applied to MDD, bipolar I, and bipolar II disorder.
- These patients experience symptoms that are predominantly confined to a specific season.
- The season is typically winter.
- Episodes of seasonal symptoms must outnumber nonseasonal episodes.
- In the 2 years prior to diagnosis, symptoms occurred only during the specific season.
- An effective adjunct to pharmacological treatment is bright-light therapy.
- The regimen of choice for bright-light therapy is 30 minutes of 10,000 lux (intensity) before 8AM.

Rapid Cycling Specifier
- Rapid cycling applies only to bipolar I and bipolar II disorder.
- These patients experience at least 4 mood disturbance episodes over the course of 1 year.
- Rapid cycling is best treated with the mood stabilizers valproate or carbamazepine (not lithium).

Chronic Specifier
- Chronic specifier can apply to MDD, bipolar I, and bipolar II disorder.
- This specifier is used when a major depressive episode lasts continuously for 2 years.

Anxiety Disorders: The Basics

IDENTIFICATION

There are 8 anxiety disorders:
1) Panic Disorder
2) Agoraphobia
3) Social Phobia
4) Specific Phobia
5) Obsessive-Compulsive Disorder
6) Posttraumatic Stress Disorder
7) Acute Stress Disorder
8) Generalized Anxiety Disorder

CHARACTERISTICS

Anxiety is characterized by:
1) excessive worry
2) fear of illness or impending doom
3) multiple somatic complaints
4) avoidant behavior of anxiety-provoking stimuli

Panic Disorder may occur with or without agoraphobia. Panic disorder is diagnosed in the presence of recurrent panic attacks. Panic attacks are discrete periods of fear or discomfort with at least 4 other panic-like symptoms.

Agoraphobia is a fear of leaving home and may occur with or without a history of panic disorder. Patients are afraid of being outside in places where escape would be difficult if panic or medical illness ensues.

Social Phobia is characterized by a fear of embarrassment in social situations where performance may be scrutinized.

Specific Phobia is characterized by fear of a specific object or situation (e.g., snakes, heights). The anticipation of that object or situation also produces anxiety.

Obsessive-Compulsive Disorder is characterized by obsessive thoughts that produce anxiety and compulsive behaviors (or mental acts) that are designed to alleviate it. Obsessions are recurrent and obtrusive thoughts or feelings and compulsions are repetitive patterns of behavior (e.g., counting or checking).

Posttraumatic Stress Disorder occurs after a person has been exposed to a severe traumatic stressor that involved the threat of death. The person then persistently re-experiences the trauma and associated symptoms of anxiety and arousal.

Acute Stress Disorder is also a post-traumatic disorder, but the associated symptoms of anxiety must occur within 4 weeks of experiencing the traumatic stressor.

Generalized Anxiety Disorder is characterized by excessive worry and anxiety for a 6-month period. The patient also experiences somatic symptoms such as muscle tension.

Anxiety Disorders: Essential Features

REVIEW

Anxiety disorders are the most common psychiatric diagnoses. Anxiety may be a symptom of many medical conditions or psychiatric disorders. It is crucial to distinguish between *normal* anxiety reactions to stress or fear and *pathological* anxiety. Normal anxiety is considered an adaptive response and pathological anxiety is an inappropriate reaction to a given stimulus. The anxiety disorders can be grouped into 5 main categories: (1) panic disorder, (2) phobias, (3) obsessive-compulsive disorder, (4) stress disorders, and (5) generalized anxiety disorder. This section will review the essential features of the anxiety disorders.

ESSENTIAL FEATURES

Panic Disorder
- Panic disorder is diagnosed after recurrent panic attacks.
- There are 13 symptoms of a panic attack, and 4 are required for diagnosis: (1) **palpitations,** (2) **sweating,** (3) **trembling** or shaking, (4) **shortness of breath,** (5) **feeling of choking,** (6) **chest pain** or discomfort, (7) **nausea,** (8) **dizziness,** (9) **derealization** or depersonalization, (10) **fear of losing control,** (11) **fear of dying,** (12) **parasthesias,** and (13) **chills** or hot flushes.
- Panic attacks are followed by at least **1 month** of concern about additional attacks, worry about the implications of the attacks (e.g., dying), or behavioral changes related to the attacks.
- Physical symptoms such as tachycardia and dyspnea may convince the patient they are about to die.
- Accompanying chest pain may cause these patients to present to the ER for fear of an MI.
- Panic attacks usually last between 5 and 20 minutes with a peak intensity at approximately 10 minutes.
- They may occur spontaneously (uncued), or follow a given stimulus (cued).
- Typical **cues** that trigger panic attacks are physical activity, excitement, psychotropic drugs, alcohol, caffeine, or phobic stimuli such as animals or elevators.
- Anticipatory anxiety of additional panic attacks may lead to **avoidant behavior** and **agoraphobia.**
- Panic disorder frequently co-exists with major depression or dysthymia.
- The onset of the disorder is typically between the ages of 20 and 30.
- Treatment requires a combination of psychotherapy and pharmacotherapy.

Agoraphobia
- Agoraphobia is a fear of leaving the safety of the home environment.
- Patients are afraid of developing symptoms of anxiety in situations where escape is difficult.
- They fear the feeling of being trapped, helpless, or embarrassed by their anxiety.
- They are also afraid to be alone and often require a companion when leaving the house.
- Typical situations that elicit fear are public transportation, crowds, elevators, and movie theatres.
- The majority of cases of agoraphobia are accompanied by panic disorder.
- Symptoms of agoraphobia usually resolve with the treatment of panic disorder.

Essential Features (continued)

Social Phobia

- Phobic disorders are the most common psychiatric diagnoses.
- Patients with social phobia are afraid of embarrassing themselves in public.
- They anticipate anxiety under **performance situations** and dread the possibility of **humiliation.**
- They typically avoid performing tasks or speaking in front of other people.
- Other social situations that elicit a phobic reaction are eating, writing, and using public restrooms.
- Physical symptoms of anxiety may be experienced; **blushing** is the most common.
- These patients can accurately identify the phobic stimuli, and describe the symptoms and avoidant behavior associated with the anxiety.
- Social phobia may be generalized or limited to specific situations (performance anxiety is the classic example of social phobia limited to specific situations).
- The disease course varies and the prognosis is dependent on the degree of functional impairment.
- Psychotherapy and pharmacotherapy are both effective treatments.

Specific Phobia

- Specific phobias are fears of certain objects and situations.
- The phobic stimuli must *always* elicit the emotional response of anxiety.
- People with a specific phobia exhibit avoidant behavior of the phobic stimuli.
- The *consequences* of encountering the phobic stimuli are what elicit the fear and anxiety.
- Examples of specific phobias are a fear of suffocation from closed spaces or being bitten by an animal.
- The DSM-IV lists 4 types of specific phobias: (1) **animal,** (2) **natural environment** (heights and storms), (3) **blood-injection** (needles and medical procedures), and (4) **situational** (planes, elevators, enclosed places).
- Treatment is usually accomplished with behavioral therapy techniques.

Obsessive-Compulsive Disorder

- Obsessive-compulsive disorder (OCD) affects 2 to 3 percent of the population.
- Obsessions are thoughts, impulses, or feelings that create anxiety in the person experiencing them.
- Compulsions are ritualistic behaviors or mental acts specifically designed to reduce anxiety.
- There are 4 main symptom patterns in obsessive-compulsive disorder: (1) contamination, (2) pathological doubt, (3) intrusive thoughts, and (4) need for symmetry.
- Fear of **contamination** is the most common symptom, and cleaning is the associated compulsion.
- Patients are afraid of germs and may incessantly wash their hands or avoid leaving the house.
- Examples of **pathological doubt** are a fear of leaving the door unlocked or the stove turned on.
- Persistent checking is the compulsion that accompanies pathological doubt.
- **Intrusive thoughts** are typically obsessions of a violent or sexual nature *without* an associated compulsion.
- **Symmetry** involves a pathological need for precision and a compulsion for slowness.
- Obsessions are persistently intrusive and experienced as **ego-dystonic** (unacceptable to the ego).
- Compulsions often require enormous amounts of time and severely impair functioning.
- OCD is seen more frequently in patients with brain injuries or Huntington's disease.
- OCD and Tourette's syndrome frequently co-exist, and symptoms overlap across the two disorders.
- The mean age of onset of OCD is approximately 20 years old.
- Patients can suffer a chronic disease course or may only experience intermittent symptom episodes.
- The treatment of choice is pharmacotherapy with serotonin reuptake inhibitors and cognitive behavioral therapy.

Essential Features (continued)

Posttraumatic Stress Disorder

- Posttraumatic stress disorder (PTSD) occurs after a life-threatening event.
- Examples of PTSD stressors include war, rape, assault, natural disasters, car accidents, and fires.
- The 3 classic features of PTSD are (1) persistent reliving of the traumatic event, (2) a constant state of hyper-arousal, and (3) avoidant behavior with emotional numbing.
- Patients **relive** the traumatic event through nightmares, daydreams, and rumination.
- **Hyperarousal** is characterized by irritability, an increased startle response, and sleep abnormalities.
- People suffering from PTSD go to extreme measures to **avoid** being reminded of the event.
- **Survivor guilt** is a common feature of PTSD after traumatic events in which others died.
- Traumatic events only result in PTSD in a small percentage of people who are vulnerable.
- Factors that increase vulnerability include personality disorders, childhood trauma, and genetic predisposition.
- PTSD may not develop until months or years after the traumatic event.
- Symptom severity may fluctuate and often increases during times of stress.
- Treatment is with psychotherapy and pharmacotherapy.

Acute Stress Disorder

- The features of acute stress disorder are identical to PTSD *except* for the timing of the traumatic event.
- The difference is that acute stress disorder lasts a maximum of 4 weeks and must occur within 4 weeks of the traumatic event.
- Acute stress disorder is more likely than PTSD to be associated with prominent dissociative symptoms.
- Approximately 80 percent of patients with acute stress disorder go on to develop PTSD.
- As opposed to acute stress disorder, PTSD may occur at any time and can last indefinitely.

Generalized Anxiety Disorder

- The main features of generalized anxiety disorder (GAD) are (1) anxiety, (2) somatic complaints, (3) autonomic hyperactivity, and (4) hyperarousal.
- **Anxiety** occurs over a 6-month period and involves excessive worry that impairs functioning.
- **Somatic complaints** common to GAD are headaches, muscular pain, and restlessness.
- **Autonomic hyperactivity** includes shortness of breath, palpitations, and sweating.
- **Hyperarousal** is manifested by an increased startle response and persistent irritability.
- The majority of patients with GAD also suffer from another psychiatric disorder (e.g., depression).
- The combination of psychotherapy and pharmacotherapy is the most effective treatment for GAD.

Anxiety Disorders: Depth and Detail

REVIEW

Anxiety disorders, particularly phobias, are the most common psychiatric diagnoses. Anxiety tends to run in families, and women are more frequently affected than men. The onset of most anxiety disorders is during late adolescence and young adulthood, but symptoms may occur at any age. This section will review important details of the anxiety disorders and present a differential diagnosis.

PANIC DISORDER

Epidemiology
- The lifetime prevalence of panic disorder is approximately 1.5 percent.
- It occurs more frequently in women.
- The onset is usually between 20 and 30 years old, but it may begin at any age.
- Panic disorder occurs more frequently in people with mitral valve prolapse.

Etiology
- **Catecholamine theory** suggests that the etiology is excessive beta-adrenergic discharge.
- **Locus ceruleus theory** views increased noradrenergic discharge as the cause of panic disorder.
- **GABA theory** suggests decreased inhibition in panic disorder due to abnormal GABA receptors.
- **CO_2 hypersensitivity theory** refers to brain stem receptor sensitivity and a resultant increase in vulnerability to panic disorder.
- **Genetic influences** are widely accepted, and panic disorder tends to run in families.

Diagnostic criteria for Panic Disorder Without Agoraphobia
And Panic Disorder With Agoraphobia

A. Both (1) and (2):
   (1) recurrent unexpected Panic Attacks
   (2) at least one of the attacks has been followed by 1 month (or more) of one (or more) of the following:
      (a) persistent concern about having additional attacks
      (b) worry about the implications of the attack or its consequences (e.g., losing control, having a heart attack, "going crazy")
      (c) a significant change in behavior related to the attacks
B. Absence of Agoraphobia (300.01); presence of Agoraphobia (300.21)
C. The Panic Attacks are not due to the direct physiological effects of a substance (e.g., a drug of abuse, a medication) or a general medical condition (e.g., hyperthyroidism).
D. The Panic Attacks are not better accounted for by another mental disorder, such as Social Phobia (e.g., occurring on exposure to feared social situations), Specific Phobia (e.g., on exposure to a specific phobic situation), Obsessive-Compulsive Disorder (e.g., on exposure to dirt in someone with an obsession about contamination), Post-traumatic Stress Disorder (e.g., in response to stimuli associated with a severe stressor), or Separation Anxiety Disorder (e.g., in response to being away from home or close relatives).

From American Psychiatric Association: Diagnostic and Statistical Manual of Mental Disorders, 4th ed. Text Revision. Washington, DC, American Psychiatric Association, 2000. With permission.

Panic Disorder (continued)

Course and Prognosis
- Panic disorder has a waxing and waning course characterized by periods of remission and relapse.
- The severity of panic attacks varies, and they may occur daily, weekly, or monthly.
- Patients may experience significant social or occupational impairment as a result of attacks.
- Patients are at an increased risk for suicide.
- Prognosis depends on symptom severity and premorbid functioning.

Treatment
- Panic disorder is treated most effectively with pharmacotherapy and psychotherapy.
- SSRIs (fluoxetine) and benzodiazepines (alprazolam) are the most frequently used medications.
- Newer antidepressants such as nefazodone and venlafaxine are also effective.
- Cognitive-behavioral therapy is the psychotherapeutic method of choice.

AGORAPHOBIA

Epidemiology
- The prevalence of agoraphobia is difficult to ascertain because patients may not seek medical attention.
- In psychiatric settings approximately 75 percent of patients with agoraphobia also have panic disorder.

Etiology
- The proposed etiologies of agoraphobia are identical to those of panic disorder.

Diagnostic criteria for Agoraphobia

A. Anxiety about being in places or situations from which escape might be difficult (or embarrassing) or in which help may not be available in the event of having an unexpected or situationally predisposed Panic Attack or panic-like symptoms. Agoraphobic fears typically involve characteristic clusters of situations that include being outside the home alone; being in a crowd or standing in a line; being on a bridge; and traveling in a bus, train, or automobile. **Note:** Consider the diagnosis of Specific Phobia if the avoidance is limited to one or only a few specific situations, or Social Phobia if avoidance is limited to social situations.

B. The situations are avoided (e.g., travel is restricted) or else are endured with marked distress or with anxiety about having a Panic Attack or panic-like symptoms, or require the presence of a companion.

C. The anxiety or phobic avoidance is not better accounted for by another mental disorder, such as Social Phobia (e.g., avoidance limited to social situations because of fear of embarrassment), Specific Phobia (e.g., avoidance limited to a single situation like elevators), Obsessive-Compulsive Disorder (e.g., avoidance of dirt in someone with an obsession about contamination), Posttraumatic Stress Disorder (e.g., avoidance of stimuli associated with a severe stressor), or Separation Anxiety Disorder (e.g., avoidance of leaving home or relatives).

From American Psychiatric Association: Diagnostic and Statistical Manual of Mental Disorders, 4th ed. Text Revision. Washington, DC, American Psychiatric Association, 2000, with permission.

Course and Prognosis
- Agoraphobia usually occurs with panic disorder and follows the same course and prognosis.
- Most cases of agoraphobia resolve with treatment of the panic disorder.
- Agoraphobia without panic disorder is more difficult to treat and may have a chronic, debilitating course.

Agoraphobia (continued)

Treatment

- Behavioral therapy is the treatment of choice for agoraphobia.
- The most effective behavioral therapy for agoraphobia is gradual exposure.
- Pharmacotherapy with SSRIs and benzodiazepines is also effective.

SOCIAL PHOBIA

Epidemiology

- Phobias are the most prevalent psychiatric disorders.
- Social phobia occurs more frequently in women.
- It usually begins during adolescence.

Etiology

- Social phobia may be related to inherited character traits of inhibition and shyness.
- Overprotective parenting styles may be an associated factor.
- It is more likely to occur in first-degree relatives.
- Performance type of social phobia is associated with increased beta-adrenergic activity.

Diagnostic criteria for Social Phobia

A. A marked and persistent fear of one or more social or performance situations in which the person is exposed to unfamiliar people or to possible scrutiny by others. The individual fears that he or she will act in a way (or show anxiety symptoms) that will be humiliating or embarrassing. **Note:** In children, there must be evidence of the capacity for age-appropriate social relationships with familiar people and the anxiety must occur in peer settings, not just in interactions with adults.

B. Exposure to the feared social situation almost invariably provokes anxiety, which may take the form of a situationally bound or situationally predisposed Panic Attack. **Note:** In children, the anxiety may be expressed by crying, tantrums, freezing, or shrinking from social situations with unfamiliar people.

C. The person recognizes that the fear is excessive or unreasonable. **Note:** In children, this feature may be absent.

D. The feared social or performance situations are avoided or else are endured with intense anxiety or distress.

E. The avoidance, anxious anticipation, or distress in the feared social or performance situation(s) interferes significantly with the person's normal routine, occupational (academic) functioning, or social activities or relationships, or there is marked distress about having the phobia.

F. In individuals under age 18 years, the duration is at least 6 months.

G. The fear or avoidance is not due to the direct physiological effects of a substance (e.g., a drug of abuse, a medication) or a general medical condition and is not better accounted for by another mental disorder (e.g., Panic Disorder With or Without Agoraphobia, Separation Anxiety Disorder, Body Dysmorphic Disorder, a Pervasive Developmental Disorder, or Schizoid Personality Disorder).

H. If a general medical condition or another mental disorder is present, the fear in Criterion A is unrelated to it, e.g., the fear is not of Stuttering, trembling in Parkinson's disease, or exhibiting abnormal eating behavior in Anorexia Nervosa or Bulimia Nervosa.

Social Phobia (continued)

Course and Prognosis
- It follows a widely variable disease course.
- Prognosis is dependent on the extent of functional impairment and severity of comorbid disorders.

Treatment
- Social phobia is treated with psychotherapy and pharmacotherapy.
- Generalized social phobia is treated with MAOIs, SSRIs, benzodiazepines, venlafaxine, and buspirone.
- Performance type social phobia is treated with beta-blockers (propranolol).
- Cognitive-behavioral therapy is the most effective type of psychotherapy.

SPECIFIC PHOBIA

Epidemiology
- Specific phobia is more common than social phobia.
- It occurs more frequently in women and the typical age of onset is 25 years old.
- Blood/injection injury type is the phobia that is more likely to develop in childhood.

Etiology
- Specific phobias develop when objects and situations get paired with the emotional response of fear.
- The response can be a result of a specific experience such as snake bite or car accident.
- Responses can also be modeled after another person's (e.g., a parent's) specific phobia.
- Blood/injection injury phobias may be caused by a strong vasovagal reflex that is usually inherited.
- Specific phobias are more likely to be seen in first-degree relatives.

Diagnostic criteria for Specific Phobia

A. Marked and persistent fear that is excessive or unreasonable, cued by the presence or anticipation of a specific object or situation (e.g., flying, heights, animals, receiving an injection, seeing blood).

B. Exposure to the phobic stimulus almost invariably provokes an immediate anxiety response, which may take the form of a situationally bound or situationally predisposed Panic Attack. **Note:** In children, the anxiety may be expressed by crying, tantrums, freezing, or clinging.

C. The person recognizes that the fear is excessive or unreasonable. **Note:** In children, this feature may be absent.

D. The phobic situation(s) is avoided or else is endured with intense anxiety or distress.

E. The avoidance, anxious anticipation, or distress in the feared situation(s) interferes significantly with the person's normal routine, occupational (or academic) functioning, or social activities or relationships, or there is marked distress about having the phobia.

F. In individuals under age 18 years, the duration is at least 6 months.

G. The anxiety, Panic Attacks, or phobic avoidance associated with the specific object or situation are not better accounted for by another mental disorder, such as Obsessive-Compulsive Disorder (e.g., fear of dirt in someone with an obsession about contamination), Posttraumatic Stress Disorder (e.g., avoidance of stimuli associated with a severe stressor), Separation Anxiety Disorder (e.g., avoidance of school), Social Phobia (e.g., avoidance of social situations because of fear of embarrassment), Panic Disorder With Agoraphobia, or Agoraphobia Without History of Panic Disorder.

From American Psychiatric Association: Diagnostic and Statistical Manual of Mental Disorders, 4th ed. Text Revision. Washington, DC, American Psychiatric Association, 2000, with permission.

Specific Phobia (continued)

Course and Prognosis

- The disease course of phobias is unclear.
- Prognosis is dependent on the degree of functional impairment.

Treatment

- The treatment of choice is behavioral therapy with a graded exposure technique.
- Hypnosis and relaxation techniques have also been used with good effect.
- Beta-blockers may be used to decrease anxiety associated with phobic stimuli.

OBSESSIVE-COMPULSIVE DISORDER

Epidemiology

- The prevalence of obsessive-compulsive disorder is approximately 2 to 3 percent of the population.
- Men and women are equally affected.
- The mean age of onset is approximately 20 years old.

Etiology

- The proposed **biochemical etiology** of OCD is a dysregulation of serotonin.
- CT and MRI studies show a bilateral decrease in the size of the caudate in patients with OCD.
- There is also a well-documented **genetic component** to OCD.
- Approximately 35 percent of first-degree relatives are also affected by OCD.
- Monozygotic twins have a higher concordance rate for OCD than dizygotic twins.
- OCD is seen more frequently after brain injuries or neurological disease such as Huntington's.
- **Behavioral theory** suggests that obsessions result from classical conditioning. Neutral stimuli become paired with emotional responses of anxiety, and compulsions are a learned pattern of behavior that becomes fixed as anxiety is reduced.

Diagnostic criteria for Obsessive-Compulsive Disorder

A. Either obsessions or compulsions:

Obsessions as defined by (1), (2), (3), and (4):

   (1) recurrent and persistent thoughts, impulses, or images that are experienced, at some time during the disturbance, as intrusive and inappropriate and that cause marked anxiety or distress

   (2) the thoughts, impulses, or images are not simply excessive worries about real-life problems

   (3) the person attempts to ignore or suppress such thoughts, impulses, or images, or to neutralize them with some other thought or action

   (4) the person recognizes that the obsessional thoughts, impulses, or images are a product of his or her own mind (not imposed from without as in thought insertion)

Compulsions are defined by (1) and (2):

   (1) repetitive behaviors (e.g., hand washing, ordering, checking) or mental acts (e.g., praying, counting, repeating words silently) that the person feels driven to perform in response to an obsession, or according to rules that must be applied rigidly

   (2) the behaviors or mental acts are aimed at preventing or reducing distress or preventing some dreaded event or situation; however, these behaviors or mental acts either are not connected in a realistic way with what they are designed to neutralize or prevent or are clearly excessive

Obsessive-Compulsive Disorder (continued)

B. At some point during the course of the disorder, the person has recognized that the obsessions or compulsions are excessive or unreasonable. **Note:** This does not apply to children.

C. The obsessions or compulsions cause marked distress, are time consuming (take more than 1 hour a day), or significantly interfere with the person's normal routine, occupational (or academic) functioning, or usual social activities or relationships.

D. If another Axis I disorder is present, the content of the obsessions or compulsions is not restricted to it (e.g., preoccupation with food in the presence of an Eating Disorder; hair pulling in the presence of Trichotillomania; concern with appearance in the presence of Body Dysmorphic Disorder; preoccupation with drugs in the presence of a Substance Use Disorder; preoccupation with having a serious illness in the presence of Hypochondriasis; preoccupation with sexual urges or fantasies in the presence of a Paraphilia; or guilty ruminations in the presence of Major Depressive Disorder).

E. The disturbance is not due to the direct physiological effects of a substance (e.g., a drug of abuse, a medication) or a general medical condition.

From American Psychiatric Association: Diagnostic and Statistical Manual of Mental Disorders, 4th ed., Text Revision. Washington, DC, American Psychiatric Association, 2000, with permission.

Course and Prognosis
- The onset of OCD may occur suddenly or after a stressful life event.
- Symptoms are often kept secret for many years before diagnosis.
- A rule of thirds applies to disease course where one third experience significant improvement in symptoms, one third have moderate improvement, and one third do not improve or deteriorate.
- Symptoms may occur episodically or on a chronic basis.
- Prognosis is related to severity of symptoms and the patient's ability to resist compulsions.
- A good prognosis is associated with sudden onset of the disorder without precipitating factors.

Treatment
- The treatment of choice for OCD is SSRIs.
- The TCA clomipramine is also commonly used.
- Behavior therapy with graded exposure and desensitization is also an effective treatment for OCD.
- Surgery is a last resort treatment and involves cingulotomy.

POSTTRAUMATIC STRESS AND ACUTE STRESS DISORDERS

Epidemiology

- The prevalence of PTSD is approximately 1 to 3 percent of the general population.
- The disorder exists with higher frequency in high-risk groups such as veterans.
- It affects men and women with equal frequency.

Etiology

- PTSD is one of three psychiatric disorders that require a specific stressor for diagnosis.
- Acute stress disorder and adjustment disorder also require a known stressor for diagnosis.
- The subjective experience of the stress is a more significant contributing factor than the objective severity in developing stress disorders.
- Childhood trauma, personality disorders, and a perceived external locus of control (as opposed to an internal) are all predisposing factors that increase vulnerability.
- Neurotransmitter imbalance and increased autonomic nervous system response to stress have also been proposed as etiologies.

Diagnostic criteria for Posttraumatic Stress Disorder

A. The person has been exposed to a traumatic event in which both of the following were present:
   (1) the person experienced, witnessed, or was confronted with an event or events that involved actual or threatened death or serious injury, or a threat to the physical integrity of self or others
   (2) the person's response involved intense fear, helplessness, or horror. **Note:** In children, this may be expressed instead by disorganized or agitated behavior
B. The traumatic event is persistently reexperienced in one (or more) of the following ways:
   (1) recurrent and intrusive distressing recollections of the event, including images, thoughts, or perceptions. **Note:** In young children, repetitive play may occur in which themes or aspects of the trauma are expressed.
   (2) recurrent distressing dreams of the event. **Note:** In children, there may be frightening dreams without recognizable content.
   (3) acting or feeling as if the traumatic event were recurring (includes a sense of reliving the experience, illusions, hallucinations, and dissociative flashback episodes, including those that occur on awakening or when intoxicated). **Note:** In young children, trauma-specific reenactment may occur.
   (4) intense psychological distress at exposure to internal or external cues that symbolize or resemble an aspect of the traumatic event
   (5) physiological reactivity on exposure to internal or external cues that symbolize or resemble an aspect of the traumatic event
C. Persistent avoidance of stimuli associated with the trauma and numbing of general responsiveness (not present before the trauma), as indicated by three (or more) of the following:
   (1) efforts to avoid thoughts, feelings, or conversations associated with the trauma
   (2) efforts to avoid activities, places, or people that arouse recollections of the trauma
   (3) inability to recall an important aspect of the trauma
   (4) markedly diminished interest or participation in significant activities
   (5) feeling of detachment or estrangement from others
   (6) restricted range of affect (e.g., unable to have loving feelings)
   (7) sense of a foreshortened future (e.g., does not expect to have a career, marriage, children, or a normal life span)

Posttraumatic Stress and Acute Stress Disorders (continued)

D. Persistent symptoms of increased arousal (not present before the trauma), as indicated by two (or more) of the following:
   (1) difficulty falling or staying asleep
   (2) irritablility or outbursts of anger
   (3) difficulty concentrating
   (4) hypervigilance
   (5) exaggerated startle response
E. Duration of the disturbance (symptoms in Criteria B, C, and D) is more than 1 month.
F. The disturbance causes clinically significant distress or impairment in social, occupational, or other important areas of functioning.

Diagnostic criteria for 308.3 Acute Stress Disorder

A. The person has been exposed to a traumatic event in which both of the following were present:
   (1) the person experienced, witnessed, or was confronted with an event or events that involved actual or threatened death or serious injury, or a threat to the physical integrity of self or others
   (2) the person's response involved intense fear, helplessness, or horror
B. Either while experiencing or after experiencing the distressing event, the individual has three (or more) of the following dissociative symptoms:
   (1) a subjective sense of numbing, detachment, or absence of emotional responsiveness
   (2) a reduction in awareness of his or her surroundings (e.g., "being in a daze")
   (3) derealization
   (4) depersonalization
   (5) dissociative amnesia (i.e., inability to recall an important aspect of the trauma)
C. The traumatic event is persistently reexperienced in at least one of the following ways: recurrent images, thoughts, dreams, illusions, flashback episodes, or a sense of reliving the experience; or distress on exposure to reminders of the traumatic event.
D. Marked avoidance of stimuli that arouse recollections of the trauma (e.g., thoughts, feelings, conversations, activities, places, people).
E. Marked symptoms of anxiety or increased arousal (e.g., difficulty sleeping, irritability, poor concentration, hypervigilance, exaggerated startle response, motor restlessness).
F. The disturbance causes clinically significant distress or impairment in social, occupational, or other important areas of functioning or impairs the individual's ability to pursue some necessary task, such as obtaining necessary assistance or mobilizing personal resources by telling family members about the traumatic experience.
G. The disturbance lasts for a minimum of 2 days and a maximum of 4 weeks and occurs within 4 weeks of the traumatic event.
H. The disturbance is not due to the direct physiological effects of a substance (e.g., a drug of abuse, a medication) or a general medical condition, is not better accounted for by Brief Psychotic Disorder, and is not merely an exacerbation of a preexisting Axis I or Axis II disorder.

From American Psychiatric Association: Diagnostic and Statistical Manual of Mental Disorders, 4th ed., Text Revision. Washington, DC, American Psychiatric Association, 2000, with permission.

Posttraumatic Stress and Acute Stress Disorders (continued)

Course and Prognosis

- PTSD may develop at any time following trauma.
- Acute stress disorder must occur within 4 weeks of the traumatic event and may not last more than 4 weeks.
- Symptoms may fluctuate in severity, and patients experience exacerbations during stressful life events.
- Rapid symptom onset in PTSD is associated with a good prognosis.
- Approximately one third of patients with PTSD recover completely.

Treatment

- Supportive psychotherapy with an emphasis on developing effective coping strategies is used.
- Drug treatment is usually with imipramine or amitriptyline for at least one year.
- SSRIs, MAOIs, trazodone, and benzodiazepines are also used.

GENERALIZED ANXIETY DISORDER

Epidemiology

- GAD is a common disorder with a prevalence of approximately 5 percent.
- It is frequently associated with other psychiatric disorders such as major depression.
- It occurs more often in women.

Etiology

- There is no accepted etiology, but proposed theories are biological and psychosocial.
- **Biological theories** include GABA deficiency and reduced sensitivity of alpha2 receptors.
- One **psychosocial theory** suggests that cognitive distortions play a significant role, in which patients focus their attention on negative details and inaccurately perceive their ability to cope.
- Stressful life events increase the possibility of developing GAD.

Diagnostic criteria for Generalized Anxiety Disorder

A. Excessive anxiety and worry (apprehensive expectation), occurring more days than not for at least 6 months, about a number of events or activities (such as work or school performance).

B. The person finds it difficult to control the worry.

C. The anxiety and worry are associated with three (or more) of the following six symptoms (with at least some symptoms present for more days than not for the past 6 months).   **Note:** Only one item is required in children.

    (1) restlessness or feeling keyed up or on edge

    (2) being easily fatigued

    (3) difficulty concentrating or mind going blank

    (4) irritability

    (5) muscle tension

    (6) sleep disturbance (difficulty falling or staying asleep, or restless unsatisfying sleep)

D. The focus of the anxiety and worry is not confined to features of an Axis I disorder, e.g., the anxiety or worry is not about having a Panic Attack (as in Panic Disorder), being embarrassed in public (as in Social Phobia), being contaminated (as in Obsessive-Compulsive Disorder), being away from home or close relatives (as in Separation Anxiety Disorder), gaining weight (as in Anorexia Nervosa), having multiple physical complaints (as in Somatization Disorder), or having a serious illness (as in Hypochondriasis), and the anxiety and worry do not occur exclusively during Posttraumatic Stress Disorder.

Generalized Anxiety Disorder (continued)

E. The anxiety, worry, or physical symptoms cause clinically significant distress or impairment in social, occupational, or other important areas of functioning.

F. The disturbance is not due to the direct physiological effects of a substance (e.g., a drug of abuse, a medication) or a general medical condition (e.g., hyperthyroidism) and does not occur exclusively during a Mood Disorder, a Psychotic Disorder, or a Pervasive Developmental Disorder.

From American Psychiatric Association: Diagnostic and Statistical Manual of Mental Disorders, 4th ed., Text Revision. Washington, DC, American Psychiatric Association, 2000, with permission.

Course and Prognosis

- Course and prognosis are dependent on comorbid psychiatric disorders.
- Approximately one quarter of patients eventually develop panic disorder or major depression.

Treatment

- The combination of psychotherapy and pharmacotherapy is the most effective treatment for GAD.
- Psychotherapy techniques include cognitive-behavioral, insight-oriented, and supportive.
- Benzodiazepines are the most common medication choice.
- SSRIs, buspirone, venlafaxine, or beta-blockers are also used.

DIFFERENTIAL DIAGNOSIS

Medical

Cardiovascular disease (myocardial infarction, angina, CHF, HTN, and mitral valve prolapse)
Respiratory disease (asthma and COPD)
Endocrine diseases (carcinoid syndrome, hypoglycemia, and hyperthyroidism)
Drug intoxication (amphetamines, marijuana, nicotine, theophylline, and hallucinogens)
Neurological disorders (epilepsy, tumors, cerebrovascular disease, and trauma)

Psychiatric

Adjustment disorder with anxiety
Hypochondriasis
Somatization disorder
Malingering
Factitious disorder
Major depression
Avoidant, obsessive-compulsive, dependent, and borderline personality disorders
Separation anxiety disorder

Personality Disorders: The Basics

IDENTIFICATION

There are 10 personality disorders that fall into 3 clusters:

Cluster A (Odd/Eccentric)
1) Paranoid
2) Schizoid
3) Schizotypal

Cluster B (Dramatic/Emotional)
1) Antisocial
2) Borderline
3) Histrionic
4) Narcissistic

Cluster C (Anxious/Fearful)
1) Avoidant
2) Dependent
3) Obsessive-compulsive

CHARACTERISTICS

All personality disorders are characterized by behavior that:
1) deviates from cultural standards
2) is rigid and pervasive
3) is consistent over time
4) causes distress or functional impairment

Paranoid Personality Disorder is characterized by distrust and suspiciousness of other people.

Schizoid Personality Disorder describes people with a pervasive detachment from social interaction.

Schizotypal Personality Disorder is characterized by bizarre behavior and ideas and a reduced capacity for social relationships.

Antisocial Personality Disorder is diagnosed in people who show a consistent pattern of disregard for the rights of others. The pattern of behavior must have been present since the age of 15.

Borderline Personality Disorder describes people who show a pervasive pattern of (1) unstable relationships, (2) unstable affect, (3) unstable self-image, and (4) unstable impulse control.

Histrionic Personality Disorder describes people who demonstrate excessive emotional expression and attention-seeking behavior.

Narcissistic Personality Disorder is characterized by a heightened sense of entitlement, exaggerated feelings of self-importance, and fragile self-esteem.

Avoidant Personality Disorder is diagnosed in people who are impaired in social interactions because of feelings of inadequacy and fear of rejection.

Dependent Personality Disorder describes people who have an excessive need to be cared for and a fear of separation.

Obsessive-Compulsive Personality Disorder is characterized by a preoccupation with orderliness and control.

Personality Disorders: Essential Features

REVIEW

Personality disorders are diagnosed on Axis II. They are often referred to as "character disorders" or "Axis II" in general. It is extremely important to distinguish between personality disorders and personality traits. Every person has traits that are consistent with personality disorders. The difference between personality disorders and personality traits lies in symptom severity and the degree of functional impairment. In order to diagnose a personality disorder the characteristic behavior must (1) deviate from cultural standards, (2) be rigid and pervasive, (3) be consistent over time, and (4) cause distress or functional impairment. This section will review the essential features of the personality disorders.

ESSENTIAL FEATURES OF CLUSTER A (ODD/ECCENTRIC)

Paranoid Personality Disorder

- These people appear **guarded** and **suspicious** and are always afraid of being deceived.
- They tend to interpret other people's actions as harmful or threatening.
- People with paranoid personality disorder are quick to anger and persistently bear grudges.
- Their affect is usually constricted and they tend to lack interpersonal warmth.
- They use **projection** as their defense mechanism, attributing their own unacceptable thoughts and impulses to others.
- **Denial** is also frequently used, where they refuse to accept or acknowledge painful aspects of reality.
- The differential diagnosis includes paranoid type schizophrenia and delusional disorder.

Schizoid Personality Disorder

- These people appear **emotionally withdrawn** and usually avoid eye contact.
- They may seem self-absorbed and cold, but they are actually afraid of intimacy.
- Unlike people with social phobia or avoidant personality disorder, people with schizoid personality disorder are not interested in relationships and **do not seek social interaction.**
- Their defense mechanism is **fantasy** where imaginary friends or lovers substitute for actual ones.
- The fantasy mechanism serves to express underlying conflicts or to obtain gratification.
- The differential diagnosis includes social phobia and avoidant and schizotypal personality disorders.

Schizotypal Personality Disorder

- People with schizotypal personality disorder are overtly **strange** and **bizarre.**
- Peculiar notions, **magical thinking,** and **ideas of reference** are characteristic of this disorder.
- Although thought disorder is absent, speech may be difficult to interpret.
- Because of **inappropriate behavior** these people are socially isolated.
- Schizotypal personality disorder is sometimes considered along the schizophrenic spectrum.
- People with schizotypal personality disorder are more likely to have a family history of schizophrenia.
- A small percentage of these people may demonstrate *brief* psychotic symptoms.
- The differential diagnosis includes schizophrenia and schizoid and avoidant personality disorders.

ESSENTIAL FEATURES OF CLUSTER B (DRAMATIC/EMOTIONAL)

Antisocial Personality Disorder (ASP)

- These people are consistently **deceitful** and **manipulative,** and without regard for other people.
- On the surface, they may appear intelligent or charming.
- Probing will reveal a history of truancy from school, fighting, illegal activity, and **impulsive** behavior.
- Antisocial behavior must have been present since the age of 15, and the person needs to be at least 18 for diagnosis.
- The diagnosis of ASP is only made if antisocial behavior is pervasive and *not* state-dependent, in other words, not exclusively associated with intoxication, mania, or psychosis.
- People with ASP make up a large percentage of the prison population.
- **Substance abuse** (particularly alcohol) is more common in these people and their families.
- Multiple somatic complaints and somatization disorder are also associated with ASP.
- There is a characteristic **lack of remorse** associated with their actions.
- There may be soft neurological signs suggesting brain damage from childhood.
- The differential diagnosis includes conduct disorder, substance abuse, and bipolar disorder (manic episode).

Borderline Personality Disorder

- The term "borderline" refers to the border between neurosis and psychosis.
- These people have **unstable relationships, unstable affect, unstable self-image,** and **poor impulse control.**
- Interpersonal relationships are characterized by a **fear of abandonment** and dependency.
- Affect is **labile** and patients may appear depressed, and then angry or euphoric a moment later.
- They complain of loneliness, feeling "empty," and lacking a sense of identity (identity diffusion).
- Their behavior is unpredictable and they may **attempt suicide** or perform self-mutilating acts.
- This disorder is often comorbid with substance abuse and major depression.
- A history of being physically or sexually abused is common in women with borderline personality disorder.
- They use **splitting** as their defense mechanism, viewing people or themselves as either "all good" or "all bad."
- People with borderline personality disorder may also alternately idealize and devalue the same person.
- Other characteristic defense mechanisms are **denial,** and **projective identification.**
- Projective identification occurs when people attribute their own unacknowledged feelings to another person, and then identify with that person for feeling the way they themselves do.
- The differential diagnosis includes mood disorders and symptoms secondary to substance abuse.

Histrionic Personality Disorder

- People with histrionic personality disorder always need to be the **center of attention.**
- Their behavior is often **seductive** and **flirtatious.**
- They tend to dress in colorful and dramatic clothing.
- They express themselves in a theatrical fashion and have **exaggerated** and **shallow emotional responses.**
- Relationships are usually viewed as more serious or intimate than they actually are.
- **Somatization disorder** and mood disorders frequently co-occur with histrionic personality disorder.
- People with histrionic personality disorder use **repression** and **dissociation** as defense mechanisms.
- Repression is the unconscious forgetting or ignoring of unpleasant feelings.
- Dissociation is the temporary modification of personal identity to avoid emotional distress.
- The differential diagnosis includes borderline personality disorder.

Narcissistic Personality Disorder

- People with narcissistic personality disorder appear **arrogant** with a heightened sense of **self-importance.**
- They are actually extremely sensitive to criticism and suffer from **low self-esteem.**
- Their feelings of self-entitlement lead them to ignore conventional rules of behavior.
- These people are incapable of showing empathy and are only concerned with selfish pursuits.
- Fragile self-esteem makes narcissistic people more susceptible to depression.
- They use **denial** and **projection** as their defense mechanisms.
- In projection, people attribute their own unacceptable feelings to others.
- The differential diagnosis includes all the Cluster B personality disorders because they frequently co-exist with narcissistic personality disorder.

ESSENTIAL FEATURES OF CLUSTER C (ANXIOUS/FEARFUL)

Avoidant Personality Disorder

- During interviews, people with avoidant personality disorder appear **shy** and **anxious.**
- They avoid social contact because they are **afraid of rejection.**
- These people differ from schizoid personality disorder because they *do* desire friendship.
- People with avoidant personality disorder become socially isolated as a result of hypersensitivity to criticism and **feelings of inadequacy.**
- These people may commonly be described as having an inferiority complex.
- Anxiety and depression are common comorbid psychiatric symptoms.
- The differential diagnosis includes schizoid personality disorder and social phobia.

Dependent Personality Disorder

- People with dependent personality disorder are passive and require others to care for them.
- They have difficulty making decisions or assuming responsibility for themselves.
- They have an urgent need to be cared for in a relationship and fear being alone.
- These people tend to exhibit clinging and submissive behavior.
- **Regression** is their defense mechanism, where they return to previous stages of development to avoid current conflict.
- In shared psychotic disorder, the person diagnosed usually has dependent personality disorder.
- The differential diagnosis includes borderline personality disorder because of the fear of abandonment.

Essential Features of Cluster C (Anxious/Fearful) (continued)

Obsessive-Compulsive Personality Disorder

- People with obsessive-compulsive personality disorder are typically inflexible perfectionists.
- They require order and control in all aspects of their lives.
- They may be unable to complete tasks due to compulsive attention to detail.
- Their relationships are often cold and rigid and they have trouble with intimacy.
- Anxiety is associated with anything that upsets the normal routine of their lives.
- Unlike most people with personality disorders, these obsessive-compulsive people recognize their symptoms and acknowledge the distress it causes them.
- The defense mechanisms these people use are **reaction formation, isolation,** and **undoing.**
- In reaction formation, people deny unacceptable feelings by adopting the opposite attitude.
- Isolation is the intrapsychic separation of an unacceptable feeling from the affect that accompanies it and the subsequent repression of the feeling.
- Undoing is where people use specific behaviors to symbolically negate unacceptable thoughts, feelings, or actions.
- The differential diagnosis includes obsessive-compulsive disorder and can be distinguished by increased symptom severity in OCD.

PERSONALITY DISORDER NOT OTHERWISE SPECIFIED (NOS)

This diagnostic category is reserved for disorders that fall short of specific criteria but still demonstrate behavior that is consistent with personality disorders in general (i.e., behavior deviates from cultural standards, is rigid and pervasive, is consistent over time, and causes distress or functional impairment). **Passive-aggressive** personality disorder and **depressive** personality disorder both fall into the NOS category.

Passive Aggressive Personality Disorder

- These people procrastinate, do not perform tasks adequately, and make excuses for their behavior.
- They manipulate themselves into dependent positions and force others to become responsible for them.
- Passive-aggressive people are pessimistic and generally lack self-confidence.
- Friends become angry and frustrated with these people and often feel manipulated.
- **Reaction formation** is their defense mechanism (denial of unacceptable feelings by adopting the opposite attitude).

Depressive Personality Disorder

- These people are chronically unhappy, anhedonic, and generally pessimistic.
- Their personality traits are consistent with depressive symptoms but they do not fully meet diagnostic criteria for MDD or dysthymia.
- Their lives are usually described as lonely and sad.
- They tend to feel hopeless and inadequate with frequent self-doubting.

Personality Disorders: Depth and Detail

REVIEW

Axis II disorders present a serious clinical challenge because patients are often resistant to treatment. Maladaptive behavior patterns were generally developed over a lifetime of interacting with the environment, and people with personality disorders consider their symptoms to be "ego-syntonic" (acceptable to the ego). They tend to minimize their symptoms and deny any associated distress or anxiety. It is also quite difficult to diagnose axis II disorders in the presence of severe Axis I pathology. This section will review the important details of the personality disorders.

CLUSTER A (ODD/ECCENTRIC)

Epidemiology

- All Cluster A diagnoses are more common in men.
- Schizoid personality disorder is the most common and occurs in approximately 7.5 percent of the general population.
- People with schizotypal personality disorder are more likely to have a family history of schizophrenia.

Etiology

- The precise etiology of personality disorders is unclear.
- Environmental *and* biological factors both contribute to their development.
- Environmental factors may include child abuse, child neglect, and inconsistent parenting.
- Biological factors are genetic diatheses or neurotransmitter imbalance.
- Biological factors play a more significant role in Cluster A disorders than in Cluster B or C disorders.
- Schizotypal personality disorder demonstrates a pattern of familial inheritance.

Diagnostic criteria for Paranoid Personality Disorder

A. A pervasive distrust and suspiciousness of others such that their motives are interpreted as malevolent, beginning by early adulthood and present in a variety of contexts, as indicated by four (or more) of the following:
  (1) suspects, without sufficient basis, that others are exploiting, harming, or deceiving him or her
  (2) is preoccupied with unjustified doubts about the loyalty or trustworthiness of friends or associates
  (3) is reluctant to confide in others because of unwarranted fear that the information will be used maliciously against him or her
  (4) reads hidden demeaning or threatening meanings into benign remarks or events
  (5) persistently bears grudges, i.e., is unforgiving of insults, injuries, or slights
  (6) perceives attacks on his or her character or reputation that are not apparent to others and is quick to react angrily or to counterattack
  (7) has recurrent suspicions, without justification, regarding fidelity of spouse or sexual partner
B. Does not occur exclusively during the course of Schizophrenia, a Mood Disorder With Psychotic Features, or another Psychotic Disorder and is not due to the direct physiological effects of a general medical condition.

Cluster A (Odd/Eccentric) (continued)

Diagnostic criteria for Schizoid Personality Disorder

A. A pervasive pattern of detachment from social relationships and a restricted range of expression of emotions in interpersonal settings, beginning by early adulthood and present in a variety of contexts, as indicated by four (or more) of the following:

(1) neither desires nor enjoys close relationships, including being part of a family

(2) almost always chooses solitary activities

(3) has little, if any, interest in having sexual experiences with another person

(4) takes pleasure in few, if any, activities

(5) lacks close friends or confidants other than first-degree relatives

(6) appears indifferent to the praise or criticism of others

(7) shows emotional coldness, detachment, or flattened affectivity

B. Does not occur exclusively during the course of Schizophrenia, a Mood Disorder With Psychotic Features, another Psychotic Disorder, or a Pervasive Developmental Disorder and is not due to the direct physiological effects of a general medical condition.

Diagnostic criteria for 301.22 Schizotypal Personality Disorder

A. A pervasive pattern of social and interpersonal deficits marked by acute discomfort with, and reduced capacity for, close relationships as well as by cognitive or perceptual distortions and eccentricities of behavior, beginning by early adulthood and present in a variety of contexts, as indicated by five (or more) of the following:

(1) ideas of reference (excluding delusions of reference)

(2) odd beliefs or magical thinking that influences behavior and is inconsistent with subcultural norms (e.g., super-stitiousness, belief in clairvoyance, telepathy, or "sixth sense"; in children and adolescents, bizarre fantasies or preoccupations)

(3) unusual perceptual experiences, including bodily illusions

(4) odd thinking and speech (e.g., vague, circumstantial, metaphorical, overelaborate, or stereotyped)

(5) suspiciousness or paranoid ideation

(6) inappropriate or constricted affect

(7) behavior or appearance that is odd, eccentric, or peculiar

(8) lack of close friends or confidants other than first-degree relatives

(9) excessive social anxiety that does not diminish with familiarity and tends to be associated with paranoid fears rather than negative judgments about self

B. Does not occur exclusively during the course of Schizophrenia, a Mood Disorder With Psychotic Features, another Psychotic Disorder, or a Pervasive Developmental Disorder.

From American Psychiatric Association: Diagnostic and Statistical Manual of Mental Disorders, 4th ed., Text Revision. Washington, DC, American Psychiatric Association, 2000, with permission.

Course and Prognosis

- Symptoms of Cluster A disorders typically begin in childhood.
- These disorders usually follow a chronic course that may be lifelong.
- A small percentage of people with Cluster A disorders eventually develop schizophrenia.
- Schizotypal personality disorder in particular is associated with an increased risk of suicide.

Cluster A (Odd/Eccentric) (continued)

Treatment

- A combination of psychotherapy and pharmacotherapy is used to manage personality disorders.
- Psychotherapeutic techniques include cognitive-behavioral therapy, psychoanalytic (insight-oriented) therapy, and group therapy.
- People with Cluster A disorders usually do not seek treatment.
- People with schizoid or schizotypal personality disorders may do well in group settings.
- Antipsychotic medication is used to treat delusional thinking and other psychotic symptoms.

CLUSTER B (DRAMATIC/EMOTIONAL)

Epidemiology

- Cluster B disorders are more common in women, except for antisocial personality disorder (ASP).
- The prevalence of Cluster B disorders ranges from 1 to 3 percent of the *general* population.
- ASP affects approximately 3 percent of *men.*
- ASP is the only Cluster B diagnosis that demonstrates familial inheritance.
- Cluster B disorders frequently co-occur with substance abuse, somatization disorder, and depression.

Etiology

- Cluster B personality disorders occur as a result of environmental and biological interaction.
- People with borderline personality disorder may have suffered from sexual or physical abuse.
- Aggressive and impulsive behavior are associated with low levels of serotonin metabolite (5-HIAA).

Diagnostic criteria for Antisocial Personality Disorder

A. There is a pervasive pattern of disregard for and violation of the rights of others occurring since age 15 years, as indicated by three (or more) of the following:
   (1) failure to conform to social norms with respect to lawful behaviors as indicated by repeatedly performing acts that are grounds for arrest
   (2) deceitfulness, as indicated by repeated lying, use of aliases, or conning others for personal profit or pleasure
   (3) impulsivity or failure to plan ahead
   (4) irritability and aggressiveness, as indicated by repeated physical fights or assaults
   (5) reckless disregard for safety of self or others
   (6) consistent irresponsibility, as indicated by repeated failure to sustain consistent work behavior or honor financial obligations
   (7) lack of remorse, as indicated by being indifferent to or rationalizing having hurt, mistreated, or stolen from another
B. The individual is at least age 18 years.
C. There is evidence of Conduct Disorder with onset before age 15 years.
D. The occurrence of antisocial behavior is not exclusively during the course of Schizophrenia or a Manic Episode.

Diagnostic criteria for Borderline Personality Disorder

A pervasive pattern of instability of interpersonal relationships, self-image, and affects, and marked impulsivity beginning by early adulthood and present in a variety of contexts, as indicated by five (or more) of the following:
(1) frantic efforts to avoid real or imagined abandonment.   **Note:** Do not include suicidal or self-mutilating behavior covered in Criterion 5.

Cluster B (Dramatic/Emotional) (continued)

(2) a pattern of unstable and intense interpersonal relationships characterized by alternating between extremes of idealization and devaluation

(3) identity disturbance: markedly and persistently unstable self-image or sense of self

(4) impulsivity in at least two areas that are potentially self-damaging (e.g., spending, sex, substance abuse, reckless driving, binge eating).   **Note:** Do not include suicidal or self-mutilating behavior covered in Criterion 5.

(5) recurrent suicidal behavior, gestures, or threats, or self-mutilating behavior

(6) affective instability due to a marked reactivity of mood (e.g., intense episodic dysphoria, irritability, or anxiety usually lasting a few hours and only rarely more than a few days)

(7) chronic feelings of emptiness

(8) inappropriate, intense anger or difficulty controlling anger (e.g., frequent displays of temper, constant anger, recurrent physical fights)

(9) transient, stress-related paranoid ideation or severe dissociative symptoms

Diagnostic criteria for Histrionic Personality Disorder

A pervasive pattern of excessive emotionality and attention seeking, beginning by early adulthood and present in a variety of contexts, as indicated by five (or more) of the following:

(1) is uncomfortable in situations in which he or she is not the center of attention

(2) interaction with others is often characterized by inappropriate sexually seductive or provocative behavior

(3) displays rapidly shifting and shallow expression of emotions

(4) consistently uses physical appearance to draw attention to self

(5) has a style of speech that is excessively impressionistic and lacking in detail

(6) shows self-dramatization, theatricality, and exaggerated expression of emotion

(7) is suggestible, i.e., easily influenced by others or circumstances

(8) considers relationships to be more intimate than they actually are

Diagnostic criteria for Narcissistic Personality Disorder

A pervasive pattern of grandiosity (in fantasy or behavior), need for admiration, and lack of empathy, beginning by early adulthood and present in a variety of contexts, as indicated by five (or more) of the following:

(1) has a grandiose sense of self-importance (e.g., exaggerates achievements and talents, expects to be recognized as superior without commensurate achievements)

(2) is preoccupied with fantasies of unlimited success, power, brilliance, beauty, or ideal love

(3) believes that he or she is "special" and unique and can only be understood by, or should associate with, other special or high-status people (or institutions)

(4) requires excessive admiration

(5) has a sense of entitlement, i.e., unreasonable expectations of especially favorable treatment or automatic compliance with his or her expectations

(6) is interpersonally exploitative, i.e., takes advantage of others to achieve his or her own ends

(7) lacks empathy: is unwilling to recognize or identify with the feelings and needs of others

(8) is often envious of others or believes that others are envious of him or her

(9) shows arrogant, haughty behaviors or attitudes

From American Psychiatric Association: Diagnostic and Statistical Manual of Mental Disorders, 4th ed., Text Revision. Washington, DC, American Psychiatric Association, 2000, with permission.

Cluster B (Dramatic/Emotional) (continued)

Course and Prognosis
- Cluster B disorders begin in adolescence.
- The course of symptoms is stable with a possibility of improvement over time.
- The prognosis depends on the patient's motivation for recovery and comorbid illness such as depression or substance abuse.

Treatment
- Management may be accomplished with psychotherapy and pharmacotherapy.
- Insight-oriented psychoanalytic psychotherapy is often used.
- Cognitive-behavioral therapy may be effective in borderline personality disorder for impulse control and reducing hypersensitivity to criticism.
- Mood stabilizers are effective in treating impulse control problems.
- Antidepressants are used for depression and somatic complaints.

CLUSTER C (ANXIOUS/FEARFUL)

Epidemiology
- All of the Cluster C diagnoses are more common in men except for dependent personality disorder.
- Avoidant personality disorder is the most prevalent.
- The prevalence rates for dependent and obsessive-compulsive personality disorders are unknown.
- Cluster C disorders often co-exist with anxiety and depression.

Etiology
- Environmental factors are more likely to play the causative role in Cluster C personality disorders.
- Specific parenting styles often contribute to their development.
- Avoidant personality disorder may be the result of hypercritical parents.
- Excessively controlling parents may cause children to develop obsessive-compulsive traits.

Diagnostic criteria for Avoidant Personality Disorder

A pervasive pattern of social inhibition, feelings of inadequacy, and hypersensitivity to negative evaluation, beginning by early adulthood and present in a variety of contexts, as indicated by four (or more) of the following:
(1) avoids occupational activities that involve significant interpersonal contact, because of fears of criticism, disapproval, or rejection
(2) is unwilling to get involved with people unless certain of being liked
(3) shows restraint within intimate relationships because of the fear of being shamed or ridiculed
(4) is preoccupied with being criticized or rejected in social situations
(5) is inhibited in new interpersonal situations because of feelings of inadequacy
(6) views self as socially inept, personally unappealing, or inferior to others
(7) is unusually reluctant to take personal risks or to engage in any new activities because they may prove embarrassing

Diagnostic criteria for Dependent Personality Disorder

A pervasive and excessive need to be taken care of that leads to submissive and clinging behavior and fears of separation, beginning by early adulthood and present in a variety of contexts, as indicated by five (or more) of the following:

(1) has difficulty making everyday decisions without an excessive amount of advice and reassurance from others
(2) needs others to assume responsibility for most major areas of his or her life
(3) has difficulty expressing disagreement with others because of fear of loss of support or approval.   **Note:** Do not include realistic fears of retribution.
(4) has difficulty initiating projects or doing things on his or her own (because of a lack of self-confidence in judgment or abilities rather than a lack of motivation or energy)
(5) goes to excessive lengths to obtain nurturance and support from others, to the point of volunteering to do things that are unpleasant
(6) feels uncomfortable or helpless when alone because of exaggerated fears of being unable to care for himself or herself
(7) urgently seeks another relationship as a source of care and support when a close relationship ends
(8) is unrealistically preoccupied with fears of being left to take care of himself or herself

Diagnostic criteria for Obsessive-Compulsive Personality Disorder

A pervasive pattern of preoccupation with orderliness, perfectionism, and mental and interpersonal control, at the expense of flexibility, openness, and efficiency, beginning by early adulthood and present in a variety of contexts, as indicated by four (or more) of the following:

(1) is preoccupied with details, rules, lists, order, organization, or schedules to the extent that the major point of the activity is lost
(2) shows perfectionism that interferes with task completion (e.g., is unable to complete a project because his or her own overly strict standards are not met)
(3) is excessively devoted to work and productivity to the exclusion of leisure activities and friendships (not accounted for by obvious economic necessity)
(4) is overconscientious, scrupulous, and inflexible about matters of morality, ethics, or values (not accounted for by cultural or religious identification)
(5) is unable to discard worn-out or worthless objects even when they have no sentimental value
(6) is reluctant to delegate tasks or to work with others unless they submit to exactly his or her way of doing things
(7) adopts a miserly spending style toward both self and others; money is viewed as something to be hoarded for future catastrophes
(8) shows rigidity and stubbornness

From American Psychiatric Association: Diagnostic and Statistical Manual of Mental Disorders, 4th ed., Text Revision. Washington, DC, American Psychiatric Association, 2000, with permission.

Cluster C (Anxious/Fearful) (continued)

Course and Prognosis
- Cluster C disorders are chronic and may be lifelong.
- Obsessive-compulsive personality disorder may follow a waxing and waning disease course.
- General functioning is usually impaired unless these people remain in protected environments.
- Depression and anxiety tend to complicate these disorders over time.
- The prognosis is variable but these patients are typically motivated to change.

Treatment
- Treatment is a combination of psychotherapy and pharmacotherapy.
- Psychotherapeutic methods include cognitive-behavioral therapy, psychoanalytic (insight-oriented) therapy, and group therapy.
- Benzodiazepines are used for anxiety.
- Antidepressants are used for depression.

Child and Adolescent Disorders: The Basics

IDENTIFICATION

The most common psychiatric diagnoses seen in children and adolescents are:

1) Conduct Disorder

2) Oppositional Defiant Disorder

3) Attention Deficit/Hyperactivity Disorder

4) Mental Retardation

5) Autistic Disorder

6) Tourette's Disorder

7) Separation Anxiety Disorder

CHARACTERISTICS

Conduct Disorder is characterized by a persistent pattern of behavior that violates social norms and ignores the rights of other people. Typical features include aggressive behavior, destruction of property, and theft.

Oppositional Defiant Disorder is a less severe form of conduct disorder characterized by disobedient and hostile behavior toward authority figures.

Attention Deficit/Hyperactivity Disorder is characterized by inattentive, hyperactive, or impulsive behavior.

Mental Retardation is defined as intellectual and general functioning that is significantly below average standards expected for the person's age. IQ test scores must be below 70.

Autistic Disorder is a pervasive developmental disorder that is characterized by impairments in reciprocal social skills, language development, and behavioral repertoire.

Tourette's Disorder is characterized by motor tics and at least 1 vocal tic. A tic is defined as an involuntary, sudden, and habitual motor movement or vocalization.

Separation Anxiety Disorder is characterized by excessive anxiety about being away from home or separated from an attachment figure. The anxiety must be *inappropriate* for the developmental age.

Child and Adolescent Disorders: Essential Features

REVIEW

Conduct disorder, oppositional defiant disorder, and attention deficit/hyperactivity disorder are the most frequent reasons for inpatient psychiatric hospitalization in children and adolescents. Mood disorders and psychotic disorders may also affect this age group, but are more commonly found in late adolescence and adulthood. The following section will discuss the essential features of the most important child and adolescent disorders.

ESSENTIAL FEATURES

Conduct Disorder
- There are 4 main categories of symptomatic behavior in conduct disorder: (1) aggression to people and animals, (2) destruction of property, (3) deceitfulness or theft, and (4) serious violations of the rules.
- **Aggression** usually involves threatening other kids, physical fights, or cruelty to animals.
- **Destruction of property** includes vandalism and fire-setting behavior.
- **Deceitfulness** can manifest as lying or trying to avoid obligations or obtain favors.
- **Rule violation** involves ignoring parental curfews, running away from home, and school truancy.
- Conduct disorder is a prerequisite for the diagnosis of antisocial personality disorder in adulthood.
- Kids with conduct disorder are more likely to use drugs, alcohol and cigarettes at an early age.
- Sexual promiscuity also occurs more frequently and they may commit sexual assault.
- Conduct disorder usually begins by age 13, but symptoms may be present as early as 3.
- Three symptoms must be present for at least 3 months, and one symptom for at least 6 months.

Oppositional Defiant Disorder (ODD)
- Children with ODD have temper tantrums and actively refuse to comply with rules.
- Their behavior is described as intentionally **annoying,** persistently **defiant,** and **hostile.**
- Features of the disorder are usually apparent inside the home, but may also occur outside.
- These kids have normal intelligence but frequently do poorly in school.
- Illegal activity and serious violations of social norms *do not* occur in ODD, and for this reason it is considered a less severe form of conduct disorder.
- ODD is more likely to develop into conduct disorder (or a mood disorder) in some cases.

Attention Deficit/Hyperactivity Disorder (ADHD)
- The main symptoms of ADHD are **inattention, impulsivity,** and **hyperactivity.**
- The symptoms of ADHD must occur in *at least two* settings (e.g., school and home) and be present before 7 years old.
- In school these children speak out of turn and frequently cause behavioral disturbances.
- They have trouble listening and following instructions.
- Distractibility impairs learning and academic performance.
- A learning disorder must first be ruled out when considering ADHD.
- At home they constantly need attention and easily become irritable and angry when neglected.
- These children will run around the house and possibly cause damage.
- Their behavior may appear aggressive or defiant.
- Mood lability is a common feature.

Essential Features (continued)

Mental Retardation

- Mental retardation is defined as intellectual *and* general functioning that is significantly below average.
- Intellectual functioning is measured by a standardized intelligence test and recorded as an intelligence quotient (IQ).
- Typical tests are the WISC-III(Wechsler Intelligence Scale for Children) and the Stanford-Binet.
- The WISC-III is for school-age children and the Stanford-Binet is for younger children who are at least 2 years old.
- Average IQ is defined as 100, and mental retardation occurs 2 standard deviations below average at 70.
- Mental retardation is classified as mild, moderate, severe, and profound.
- Features need to be divided according to the degree of mental retardation.
- All people with mental retardation may demonstrate **low frustration tolerance, hyperactivity, aggression, self-injurious behavior,** and **affective instability.**

Mild (IQ of 50 to 70)

- Approximately 85 percent of people with mental retardation are categorized as mild.
- These children can succeed in special education programs.
- Social and occupational functioning is mildly impaired.
- They hold jobs, support themselves and live on their own with assistance.

Moderate (IQ of 35 to 50)

- Moderate mental retardation becomes apparent earlier than does mild.
- These children are considered trainable but only simple tasks can be accomplished.
- Communication skills do not develop adequately and social isolation results.
- Occupational and self-reliance tasks are achieved only with supervision.

Severe (IQ of 20 to 35)

- Speech and motor development are poor.
- Self-care may be possible through behavioral training.
- An institutional setting is usually required for management.

Profound (IQ of less than 20)

- Language may not exist and motor skills are severely impaired.
- Lifelong constant supervision and nursing care are required.

Autistic Disorder

- Autism is a **pervasive developmental disorder** and it must be considered on a spectrum of severity.
- Children with autism may appear very different from each other despite carrying the same diagnosis.
- Autism usually becomes apparent by the age of 3.
- The three main symptoms of autism are **impaired social interaction, delayed (or absent) language development,** and a **restricted behavioral repertoire.**
- Approximately 75 percent of people with autism also suffer from **mental retardation.**
- Children are not socially connected or interested in their surroundings.
- Abnormal eye contact is a common finding.
- Nonverbal communication often fails to develop.
- Delayed or absent *expressive* language development may be the first sign of autism.
- The first step in evaluating non-verbal children should be audiometry to rule out deafness.

Essential Features (continued)

- Activities and play of autistic children are rigid and repetitive.
- Exploratory play is minimal and lacks imagination and creativity.
- Children with autism are often inflexible in their adherence to specific routines.
- They may display a persistent preoccupation with parts of objects (e.g., metal).
- Repetitive motor mannerisms such as hand flapping, twisting, and rocking are common.
- The 3 other pervasive developmental disorders are Rett's Disorder, Childhood Disintegrative Disorder, and Asperger's Disorder.
- **Rett's Disorder** has the *clinical triad* of impaired social interaction, delayed language development, and restricted behavioral repertoire, but occurs exclusively in **girls.**
- **Childhood Disintegrative Disorder** is characterized by normal development until 2 years old, followed by a loss of previously acquired skills and development of the clinical triad.
- **Asperger's Disorder** is characterized by *normal* language development with impaired social interaction and a restricted behavioral repertoire.

Tourette's Disorder

- Tourette's disorder consists of multiple **motor tics** and at least 1 **vocal tic** for 1 year.
- The disorder usually begins between 6 and 10 years old with motor tics.
- Vocal tics typically develop several years after the initial motor tics.
- Motor tics start in the neck and face and move downward to affect the extremities over time.
- Facial tics are the most common and examples are blinking, raising eyebrows, and tongue extrusion.
- Other motor tics include neck twisting, shrugging shoulders, hand clenching, and shaking.
- Vocal tics include barking, grunting, belching, and eventually verbal shouts or coprolalia.
- Attention deficit and obsessive compulsive disorder frequently co-occur with Tourette's disorder.
- Prodromal symptoms of ADHD may appear before the onset of Tourette's disorder.

Separation Anxiety Disorder

- There are 8 symptoms of separation anxiety disorder and 3 are required for diagnosis.
- (1) Children demonstrate excessive distress when separated from home.
- (2) They are persistently worried about harm befalling an attachment figure.
- (3) They are persistently worried about losing an attachment figure.
- (4) These children are reluctant, or altogether refuse, to attend school.
- (5) There is an excessive fear of being alone or at any distance from attachment figure.
- (6) They can not sleep away from home or without the attachment figure within close proximity.
- (7) Repeated nightmares of separation are common.
- (8) Physical symptoms such as nausea and vomiting occur upon separation from attachment figure.
- Symptoms must last at least 4 weeks.
- There is often a history of separation due to illness, divorce, or death.
- Infants ($<$ 1yr) show a developmentally normal form of separation anxiety called *stranger* anxiety.
- Separation anxiety can also be considered normal in a child first beginning school.

Child and Adolescent Disorders: Depth and Detail

REVIEW

This section will review significant details relevant to child and adolescent disorders in addition to the differential diagnosis.

CONDUCT DISORDER

Epidemiology

- Conduct disorder is a common psychiatric diagnosis, particularly in the inpatient population.
- The disorder occurs more frequently in boys.
- It often co-exists with attention deficit/hyperactivity disorder, learning disorders, and depression.
- Alcohol dependence and antisocial personality disorder are more likely to be present in the *parents*.

Etiology

- Psychosocial and socioeconomic factors play a significant causative role.
- Parenting styles that are strict, punitive, or aggressive contribute to its development.
- Marital discord is common, and these kids may have initially been unwanted or unplanned pregnancies.
- Child abuse and exposure to domestic violence is more likely to occur in families of children with conduct disorder.
- Aggressive and violent behavior may be associated with *decreased* serotonin metabolite (5-HIAA) in the CSF and *increased* blood serotonin levels.

Diagnostic criteria for Conduct Disorder

A. A repetitive and persistent pattern of behavior in which the basic rights of others or major age-appropriate societal norms or rules are violated, as manifested by the presence of three (or more) of the following criteria in the past 12 months, with at least one criterion present in the past 6 months:

Aggression to people and animals

(1) often bullies, threatens, or intimidates others

(2) often initiates physical fights

(3) has used a weapon that can cause serious physical harm to others (e.g., a bat, brick, broken bottle, knife, gun)

(4) has been physically cruel to people

(5) has been physically cruel to animals

(6) has stolen while confronting a victim (e.g., mugging, purse snatching, extortion, armed robbery)

(7) has forced someone into sexual activity

Destruction of property

(8) has deliberately engaged in fire setting with the intention of causing serious damage

(9) has deliberately destroyed others' property (other than by fire setting)

Deceitfulness or theft

(10) has broken into someone else's house, building, or car

(11) often lies to obtain goods or favors or to avoid obligations (i.e., "cons" others)

(12) has stolen items of nontrivial value without confronting a victim (e.g., shoplifting, but without breaking and entering; forgery)

Conduct Disorder (continued)

Serious violations of rules

(13) often stays out at night despite parental prohibitions, beginning before age 13 years

(14) has run away from home overnight at least twice while living in parental or parental surrogate home (or once without returning for a lengthy period)

(15) is often truant from school, beginning before age 13 years

B. The disturbance in behavior causes clinically significant impairment in social, academic, or occupational functioning.

C. If the individual is age 18 years or older, criteria are not met for Antisocial Personality Disorder.

From American Psychiatric Association: Diagnostic and Statistical Manual of Mental Disorders, 4th ed., Text Revision. Washington, DC, American Psychiatric Association, 2000, with permission.

Course and Prognosis

- Conduct disorder usually begins before the age of 13 and may occur in children as young as 3.
- The symptoms develop slowly over time.
- Kids are at an increased risk for substance abuse and antisocial personality disorders in adulthood.
- Prognosis is dependent on the severity and frequency of symptomatic behavior, age of onset, and intellectual functioning.

Treatment

- Treatment settings must have consistent rules and predictable consequences for breaking the rules.
- The family environment needs to be addressed and parents should be trained in techniques that facilitate appropriate behavior.
- School counselors and teachers should be informed and encourage compliance with treatment plan.
- Medications can include low-dose antipsychotics or mood stabilizers for aggression.
- SSRIs are used for impulsivity and irritability.
- Recent studies suggest that clonidine (A2 agonist) may decrease aggressive behavior.

OPPOSITIONAL DEFIANT DISORDER

Epidemiology

- In early childhood, oppositional defiant behavior may be considered normal, or age-appropriate.
- The disorder usually begins by age 8, but can be considered at age 3.
- ODD is more common in girls *before* puberty and in boys *after* puberty.

Etiology

- ODD is considered a pathological extension of normal development.
- Children rebel against authority in an effort to establish their own autonomy.
- Environmental stressors such as trauma or illness may trigger the development of ODD.

Diagnostic criteria for Oppositional Defiant Disorder

A. A pattern of negativistic, hostile, and defiant behavior lasting at least 6 months, during which four (or more) of the following are present:

(1) often loses temper

(2) often argues with adults

(3) often actively defies or refuses to comply with adults' requests or rules

(4) often deliberately annoys people

(5) often blames others for his or her mistakes or misbehavior

(6) if often touchy or easily annoyed by others

(7) if often angry and resentful

(8) is often spiteful or vindictive

Note: Consider a criterion met only if the behavior occurs more frequently than is typically observed in individuals of comparable age and developmental level.

B. The disturbance in behavior causes clinically significant impairment in social, academic, or occupational functioning.

C. The behaviors do not occur exclusively during the course of a Psychotic or Mood Disorder.

D. Criteria are not met for Conduct Disorder, and, if the individual is age 18 years or older, criteria are not met for Antisocial Personality Disorder.

From American Psychiatric Association: Diagnostic and Statistical Manual of Mental Disorders, 4th ed., Text Revision. Washington, DC, American Psychiatric Association, 2000, with permission.

Course and Prognosis

- Course and prognosis are dependent mostly on the severity of symptoms.
- Symptom duration and comorbid disorders also affect the prognosis.

Treatment

- The treatment of choice is individual psychotherapy.
- Behavior therapy with positive reinforcement is also effective.
- Counseling and child management training are recommended for the family.

ATTENTION DEFICIT/HYPERACTIVITY DISORDER

Epidemiology

- ADHD is estimated to affect up to 10 percent of school-age boys.
- The disorder is significantly more common in boys (particularly first-born).
- The majority (>50%) of inpatients on a child psychiatric unit will carry the diagnosis of ADHD.

Etiology

- The cause of ADHD is unknown, but genetic, biochemical, and psychosocial factors contribute.
- Concordance rates are higher among monozygotic twins than dizygotic twins.
- Noradrenergic dysfunction may play a role in which an accumulation of epinephrine in the *peripheral* system may inhibit *central* epinephrine release through feedback mechanisms.
- Psychosocial deprivation and intrafamily conflict contribute to symptoms of ADHD.

Attention Deficit/Hyperactivity Disorder (continued)

Diagnostic criteria for Attention-Deficit/Hyperactivity Disorder

A. Either (1) or (2):

  (1) six (or more) of the following symptoms of **inattention** have persisted for at least 6 months to a degree that is maladaptive and inconsistent with developmental level:

  Inattention

  (a) often fails to give close attention to details or makes careless mistakes in schoolwork, work, or other activities

  (b) often has difficulty sustaining attention in tasks or play activities

  (c) often does not seem to listen when spoken to directly

  (d) often does not follow through on instructions and fails to finish school-work, chores, or duties in the workplace (not due to oppositional behavior or failure to understand instructions)

  (e) often has difficulty organizing tasks and activities

  (f) often avoids, dislikes, or is reluctant to engage in tasks that require sustained mental effort (such as school-work or homework)

  (g) often loses things necessary for tasks or activities (e.g., toys, school assignments, pencils, books, or tools)

  (h) is often easily distracted by extraneous stimuli

  (i) if often forgetful in daily activities

  (2) six (or more) of the following symptoms of **hyperactivity-impulsivity** have persisted for at least 6 months to a degree that is maladaptive and inconsistent with developmental level:

  Hyperactivity

  (a) often fidgets with hands or feet or squirms in seat

  (b) often leaves seat in classroom or in other situations in which remaining seated is expected

  (c) often runs about or climbs excessively in situations in which it is inappropriate (in adolescents or adults, may be limited to subjective feelings of restlessness)

  (d) often has difficulty playing or engaging in leisure activities quietly

  (e) is often "on the go" or often acts as if "driven by a motor"

  (f) often talks excessively

  Impulsivity

  (g) often blurts out answers before questions have been completed

  (h) often has difficulty awaiting turn

  (i) often interrupts or intrudes on others (e.g., butts into conversations or games)

B. Some hyperactive-impulsive or inattentive symptoms that caused impairment were present before age 7 years.

C. Some impairment from the symptoms is present in two or more settings (e.g., at school [or work] and at home).

D. There must be clear evidence of clinically significant impairment in social, academic, or occupational functioning.

E. The symptoms do not occur exclusively during the course of a Pervasive Developmental Disorder, Schizophrenia, or other Psychotic Disorder and are not better accounted for by another mental disorder (e.g., Mood Disorder, Anxiety Disorder, Dissociative Disorder, or a Personality Disorder).

From American Psychiatric Association: Diagnostic and Statistical Manual of Mental Disorders, 4th ed., Text Revision. Washington, DC, American Psychiatric Association, 2000, with permission.

Attention Deficit/Hyperactivity Disorder (continued)

Course and Prognosis

- ADHD is usually apparent before 7 years old.
- It is no longer considered exclusively a disorder of childhood and adolescence.
- Symptoms may remit spontaneously as the patient ages, or persist into adulthood with reduced severity.
- Hyperactivity is usually the *first* symptom to remit and is the most likely to disappear.
- These patients are at increased risk for mood disorders, substance abuse, and learning disorders.
- Prognosis is dependent on comorbid disorders, social functioning, and family dynamics.

Treatment

- CNS stimulants are the treatment of choice for ADHD–methylphenidate (Ritalin), dextroamphetamine (Dexedrine), amphetamine/dextroamphetamine (Adderall), and pemoline (Cylert).
- Clonidine (A2 agonist) is useful in treating hyperactivity.
- SSRIs can be used to treat impulsive behavior.
- Antipsychotics target aggressive behavior.
- Behavior modification and individual psychotherapy are also required as adjunctive treatment.
- Counseling and behavior management training is recommended for parents.

MENTAL RETARDATION

Epidemiology

- Mental retardation affects approximately 1 percent of the population.

Etiology

- Mental retardation may be caused by chromosomal abnormalities, inborn errors of metabolism, prenatal infection, prenatal exposure to toxins such as drugs and alcohol, and perinatal trauma.
- Approximately two thirds of people with mental retardation have an identifiable cause.
- Down's syndrome is the most common cause of mental retardation.
- Fragile X syndrome is the most common cause that is *heritable.*

Diagnostic criteria for Mental Retardation

A. Significantly subaverage intellectual functioning: an IQ of approximately 70 or below on an individually administered IQ test (for infants, a clinical judgment of significantly subaverage intellectual functioning).

B. Concurrent deficits or impairments in present adaptive functioning (i.e., the person's effectiveness in meeting the standards expected for his or her age by his or her cultural group) in at least two of the following areas: communication, self-care, home living, social/interpersonal skills, use of community resources, self-direction, functional academic skills, work, leisure, health, and safety.

C. The onset is before age 18 years.

From American Psychiatric Association: Diagnostic and Statistical Manual of Mental Disorders, 4th ed., Text Revision. Washington, DC, American Psychiatric Association, 2000, with permission.

Mental Retardation (continued)

Course and Prognosis
- The more severe the mental retardation, the earlier it is detected.
- Intellectual functioning does not improve but general functioning can.
- Improvement in general functioning is dependent on the extent of environmental support.
- Prognosis depends on the underlying disorder that caused the mental retardation.
- Severe and profound mental retardation is often associated with premature death.

Treatment
- The best treatment for mental retardation is primary prevention with good prenatal care.
- Psychoeducation and family counseling are imperative.
- Pharmacological treatment is used for associated symptoms (hyperactivity, aggression, self-injurious behavior, and affective instability).

AUTISTIC DISORDER

Epidemiology
- Autism occurs at a rate of approximately 1 case per 1,000 children.
- The rate of autism among siblings is 50 times greater than in the general population.
- It is found more frequently in boys.
- Autism is associated with Tuberous Sclerosis, Fragile X syndrome, Rubella, and Phenylketonuria.
- Autism is the most common pervasive developmental disorder.

Etiology
- Autism was first considered a psychosocial disorder related to parenting styles.
- Initial studies noted that parents of children with autism were "cold" and "disinterested."
- More recently, evidence of neurobiological components has accumulated.
- Children with autism show increased evidence of perinatal complications.
- There is growing evidence of cerebral abnormalities that may reflect **impaired cell migration** in the first six months of gestation:
- The concordance rate among monozygotic twins is approximately 36 percent.

Diagnostic criteria for Autistic Disorder

A. A total of six (or more) items from (1), (2), and (3), with at least two from (1), and one each from (2) and (3):
   (1) qualitative impairment in social interaction, as manifested by at least two of the following:
      (a) marked impairment in the use of multiple nonverbal behaviors such as eye-to-eye gaze, facial expression, body postures, and gestures to regulate social interaction
      (b) failure to develop peer relationships appropriate to developmental level
      (c) a lack of spontaneous seeking to share enjoyment, interests, or achievements with other people (e.g., by a lack of showing, bringing, or pointing out objects of interest)
      (d) lack of social or emotional reciprocity
   (2) qualitative impairments in communication as manifested by at least one of the following.
      (a) delay in, or total lack of, the development of spoken language (not accompanied by an attempt to compensate through alternative modes of communication such as gesture or mime)
      (b) in individuals with adequate speech, marked impairment in the ability to initiate or sustain a conversation with others

Autistic Disorder (continued)

      (c) stereotyped and repetitive use of language or idiosyncratic language

      (d) lack of varied, spontaneous make-believe play or social imitative play appropriate to developmental level

  (3) restricted repetitive and stereotyped patterns of behavior, interests, and activities, as manifested by at least one of the following:

      (a) encompassing preoccupation with one or more stereotyped and restricted patterns of interest that is abnormal either in intensity or focus

      (b) apparently inflexible adherence to specific, nonfunctional routines or rituals

      (c) stereotyped and repetitive motor mannerisms (e.g., hand or finger flapping or twisting, or complex whole-body movements)

      (d) persistent preoccupation with parts of objects

B. Delays or abnormal functioning in at least one of the following areas, with onset prior to age 3 years: (1) social interaction, (2) language as used in social communication, or (3) symbolic or imaginative play.

C. The disturbance is not better accounted for by Rett's Disorder for Childhood Disintegrative Disorder.

From American Psychiatric Association: Diagnostic and Statistical Manual of Mental Disorders, 4th ed., Text Revision. Washington, DC, American Psychiatric Association, 2000, with permission.

Course and Prognosis

- Autism becomes apparent in most cases before 3 years' of age and has a lifelong chronic course.
- Prognosis is related to language development and the degree of mental retardation.
- Most children demonstrate some improvement in communication and social interaction over time.
- Children with autism are more likely to demonstrate aggressive or self-mutilating behavior in late childhood or adolescence.
- Approximately one-third of people with autism may develop a seizure disorder.

Treatment

- The treatment of autism focuses on reducing odd behavioral symptoms and encouraging socially acceptable behavior.
- The development of verbal and nonverbal communication is always a goal.
- The current treatment of choice is educational methods combined with behavioral training.
- A structured classroom setting with daily rigorous behavioral training is preferred.
- Psychoeducation and support for families of children with autism is imperative.
- Haloperidol and risperidone are used to treat aggressive tendencies and self-mutilating behavior.
- SSRIs are used to decrease compulsive ritualistic behavior and repetitive movements.
- The therapeutic effect of multisensory modalities such as auditory and sensory integration training is currently being evaluated.

TOURETTE'S DISORDER

Epidemiology

- There are approximately 5 cases of Tourette's disorder per 10,000 people.
- It occurs more frequently in boys.
- Obsessive-compulsive disorder and ADHD frequently co-exist with Tourette's.

Tourette's Disorder (continued)

Etiology

- Genetic and biochemical factors are responsible for the development of Tourette's.
- There is a significantly higher prevalence among monozygotic twins.
- Tourette's disorder and tics in general are more likely to follow patterns of familial inheritance.
- Increased central dopaminergic activity has also been proposed as a causative factor.

Diagnostic criteria for Tourette's Disorder

A. Both multiple motor and one or more vocal tics have been present at some time during the illness, although not necessarily concurrently. (A *tic* is a sudden, rapid, recurrent, nonrhythmic, stereotyped motor movement or vocalization.)

B. The tics occur many times a day (usually in bouts) nearly every day or intermittently throughout a period of more than 1 year, and during this period there was never a tic-free period of more than 3 consecutive months.

C. The onset is before age 18 years.

D. The disturbance is not due to the direct physiological effects of a substance (e.g., stimulants) or a general medical condition (e.g., Huntington's disease or postviral encephalitis).

From American Psychiatric Association: Diagnostic and Statistical Manual of Mental Disorders, 4th ed., Text Revision. Washington, DC, American Psychiatric Association, 2000, with permission.

Course and Prognosis

- Tourette's is a chronic lifelong disorder with a waxing and waning course.
- Symptoms typically begin between 6 and 10 years old.
- Many comorbid psychiatric disorders may occur with Tourette's (OCD, ADHD, and MDD).
- Symptom severity and medication compliance determine the course and prognosis of the disorder.
- Some patients become socially isolated and may attempt suicide.
- Other patients are managed well with treatment.

Treatment

- Pharmacotherapy is the treatment of choice for Tourette's disorder.
- Antipsychotics, particularly haloperidol, are the most commonly prescribed medication.
- The vast majority of patients respond favorably.
- Comorbid disorders must also be appropriately treated.

SEPARATION ANXIETY DISORDER

Epidemiology

- Approximately 3 to 4 percent of children and 1 percent of adolescents are affected.
- It most commonly occurs in children 7 to 8 years old.
- It is equally prevalent in boys and girls.

Etiology

- Separation anxiety disorder has similar etiological components as other anxiety disorders.
- It is caused by a combination of inherited traits and environmental stressors.
- The biological trait of extreme shyness is considered the main contributing factor.
- The nature of the relationship and attachment to the child's mother also play a role.
- Maternal anxiety and overprotective parents increase the risk of developing separation anxiety.
- Environmental stressors include changing schools, illness, and a death in the family.

Diagnostic criteria for Separation Anxiety Disorder

A. Developmentally inappropriate and excessive anxiety concerning separation from home or from those to whom the individual is attached, as evidenced by three (or more) of the following:

   (1) recurrent excessive distress when separation from home or major attachment figures occurs or is anticipated

   (2) persistent and excessive worry about losing, or about possible harm befalling, major attachment figures

   (3) persistent and excessive worry that an untoward event will lead to separation from a major attachment figure (e.g., getting lost or being kidnapped)

   (4) persistent reluctance or refusal to go to school or elsewhere because of fear of separation

   (5) persistently and excessively fearful or reluctant to be alone or without major attachment figures at home or without significant adults in other settings

   (6) persistent reluctance or refusal to go to sleep without being near a major attachment figure or to sleep away from home

   (7) repeated nightmares involving the theme of separation

   (8) repeated complaints of physical symptoms (such as headaches, stomachaches, nausea, or vomiting) when separation from major attachment figures occurs or is anticipated

B. The duration of the disturbance is at least 4 weeks.

C. The onset is before age 18 years.

D. The disturbance causes clinically significant distress or impairment in social, academic (occupational), or other important areas of functioning.

E. The disturbance does not occur exclusively during the course of a Pervasive Developmental Disorder, Schizophrenia, or other Psychotic Disorder and, in adolescents and adults, is not better accounted for by Panic Disorder With Agoraphobia.

From American Psychiatric Association: Diagnostic and Statistical Manual of Mental Disorders, 4th ed., Text Revision. Washington, DC, American Psychiatric Association, 2000, with permission.

Course and Prognosis

- Most children who suffer from separation anxiety disorder recover within one year.
- A prolonged course increases the risk of later developing an anxiety disorder—panic disorder in particular.
- Course and prognosis are dependent on the age of onset and symptom duration.
- Children who maintain general functioning and attend school have a better prognosis.

Treatment

- A combination of psychotherapy and pharmacotherapy is the treatment of choice.
- Family psychoeducation and family therapy are also recommended.
- Individual psychotherapy and cognitive-behavioral therapy are used for the patient.
- SSRIs or benzodiazepines are usually prescribed.
- Propranolol and buspirone can also be used.
- Benadryl is effective for anxiety-related insomnia.

DIFFERENTIAL DIAGNOSIS

Conduct Disorder

Normal oppositional behavior
Oppositional defiant disorder
ADHD
Learning disorders
Substance abuse
Mental retardation

Oppositional Defiant Disorder

Normal oppositional behavior
Conduct disorder
ADHD
Learning disorders
Mental retardation

Attention Deficit/Hyperactivity Disorder

Learning disorders
Mental retardation
Anxiety disorder
Conduct disorder

Mental Retardation

Deafness
Cerebral palsy
Pervasive developmental disorders
Brain damage
Seizure disorder

Autistic Disorder

Other pervasive developmental disorders (Rett's, Asperger's, and Childhood Disintegrative Disorder)
Schizophrenia with childhood onset
Congenital deafness
Mixed receptive-expressive language disorder
Psychosocial deprivation
Mental retardation (with behavioral symptoms)
Selective mutism

Tourette's Disorder

Medication side effect (e.g., CNS stimulants for ADHD)
Huntington's disease
Sydenham's chorea
Wilson's disease
Pervasive developmental disorders
Motor compulsions

Separation Anxiety Disorder

Stranger anxiety
Normal separation anxiety
Generalized anxiety disorder
Major depression

Eating Disorders: The Basics

IDENTIFICATION

There are 2 eating disorders:

1) Anorexia Nervosa

2) Bulimia Nervosa

CHARACTERISTICS

Eating disorders are characterized by:

1) Disturbed eating behavior
2) Preoccupation with food
3) Distorted body image

Anorexia Nervosa is characterized by the refusal to maintain normal body weight. There is an intense fear of gaining weight accompanied by a distorted body image. In post-menarchal women, amenorrhea is required for diagnosis.

Bulimia Nervosa is characterized by recurrent episodes of binge eating. Symptoms may overlap with anorexia nervosa, but most patients with bulimia nervosa maintain normal body weight.

Eating Disorders: Essential Features

REVIEW

Anorexia nervosa and bulimia nervosa are both characterized by **abnormal eating behavior, excessive concern about body weight,** and a **distorted body image.** Anorexia nervosa can be distinguished from bulimia nervosa by ideal body weight. If a patient's weight falls below 85 percent of ideal body weight, the diagnosis of anorexia nervosa is made. Patients with bulimia nervosa *may* be overweight or underweight, but *most* maintain normal body weight. This section will review the essential features of the eating disorders.

ESSENTIAL FEATURES

Anorexia Nervosa

- The hallmark of the anorexia nervosa is an **intense fear of gaining weight.**
- These patients refuse to maintain a minimally normal body weight (85 percent of ideal).
- They lose weight by drastically reducing their total food intake but an actual loss of appetite does not occur until late in the disease.
- Body image is grossly distorted, and patients are convinced they appear overweight despite being significantly *below* their ideal body weight.
- There are two clinical subtypes of anorexia nervosa: restricting type and binge eating/purging type.
- In the restricting type, patients often refuse to eat, particularly with their families or in public places.
- In the purging type, eating is followed by induced vomiting, laxatives, or excessive exercise.
- In post-menarchal females, the absence of at least 3 consecutive menstrual cycles (amenorrhea) is required for diagnosis.
- When patients with anorexia nervosa do eat, it is accompanied by peculiar behavior such as cutting meat into tiny pieces and spending a lot of time arranging food on their plate.
- Anorexia nervosa may be accompanied by **compulsive behavior** revolving around food, **depression,** and **anxiety.**
- Physical signs of profound weight loss are **hypothermia, edema, bradycardia, hypotension,** and the appearance of fine, soft, neonatal-like **hair (lanugo).**
- Mortality may be as high as 18 percent and is usually secondary to medical complications or suicide.
- Medical complications include electrolyte imbalance, dehydration, and esophageal and gastric erosion.
- Patients with anorexia nervosa may be resistant to treatment and require inpatient hospitalization.
- The first goal of treatment is to stabilize the patient medically.
- After stabilization, nutritional status is restored using supervised meals and weight monitoring.

Essential Features (continued)

Bulimia Nervosa

- Bulimia nervosa is characterized by **binge eating** and **compensatory behavior** to avoid weight gain.
- There are 2 clinical subtypes of bulimia nervosa: purging type and nonpurging type.
- In purging type, patients induce vomiting and abuse laxatives, diuretics, and enemas.
- In nonpurging type bulimia nervosa, patients use fasting and exercise to counter binge eating.
- Despite compensatory behavior to avoid weight gain, these patients tend to maintain their body weight.
- Menstrual abnormalities may occur in bulimia nervosa, but are not required for diagnosis.
- Body shape and weight overwhelmingly influence their self-evaluation.
- Patients with bulimia nervosa commonly report feeling a lack of control over symptoms.
- They are often angry and impulsive and have difficulty controlling their behavior in general.
- Substance abuse and promiscuous sexual behavior often occus in bulimia nervosa.
- Bulimia nervosa has a waxing and waning course and the prognosis is usually better than in anorexia.
- Complications of purging behavior include electrolyte abnormalities, esophagitis, and dental erosion.
- Treatment is usually a combination of psychotherapy and pharmacotherapy.

Eating Disorders: Depth and Detail

REVIEW

Anorexia nervosa and bulimia nervosa occur most commonly in young women. Difficulty in adapting to adolescence and the importance that society places on thinness play indisputable roles in the development of eating disorders. Unstable family relationships and marital conflicts are also likely to affect patients with eating disorders. This section will review the important details of the eating disorders, including proposed etiologies, treatment, and the differential diagnosis.

ANOREXIA NERVOSA

Epidemiology
- Anorexia nervosa affects 0.5 to 1 percent of adolescent girls.
- It is significantly more common in women than men (10–20:1).

Etiology
- Young people with anorexia nervosa may be having difficulty adjusting to adolescence.
- They often lack a sense of autonomy and feel overly controlled by their parents.
- Self-starvation is an effort to *control* their bodies and to be recognized as independent.
- Symptoms may also serve to focus attention away from dysfunctional family relationships.
- Patients tend to be high achievers and may view starvation as an act of self-discipline.

Diagnostic criteria for Anorexia Nervosa

A. Refusal to maintain body weight at or above a minimally normal weight for age and height (e.g., weight loss leading to maintenance of body weight less that 85% of that expected; or failure to make expected weight gain during period of growth, leading to body weight less that 85% of that expected).
B. Intense fear of gaining weight or becoming fat, even though underweight.
C. Disturbance in the way in which one's body weight or shape is experienced, undue influence of body weight or shape on self-evaluation, or denial of the seriousness of the current low body weight.
D. In postmenarcheal females, amenorrhea, i.e., the absence of at least three consecutive menstrual cycles. (A woman is considered to have amenorrhea if her periods occur only following hormone, e.g., estrogen, administration.)

From American Psychiatric Association: Diagnostic and Statistical Manual of Mental Disorders, 4th ed., Text Revision. Washington, DC, American Psychiatric Association, 2000, with permission.

Course and Prognosis
- The course of anorexia nervosa is highly variable.
- Few patients recover spontaneously and some have a gradually deteriorating course resulting in death.
- Recovery may require many different treatments and only occur after several relapses.
- Mortality rates of *up to* 18 percent have been reported secondary to medical complications or suicide.
- Medical complications of eating disorders are related to weight loss and purging activity.
- **Weight loss complications** include hypothermia, cardiac arrhythmias, amenorrhea, lanugo hair, edema, leukopenia, and osteoporosis.
- **Purging activity complications** include electrolyte imbalance, dehydration, esophageal and gastric erosion or rupture, seizures, dental erosion, cognitive dysfunction, neuropathies, and ipecac toxicity.

Anorexia Nervosa (continued)

Treatment

- Patients with anorexia nervosa are extremely secretive about their symptoms and resistant to treatment.
- Patients who are below 20 percent of ideal body weight require hospitalization.
- Therapeutic intervention is not attempted until the patient is stabilized medically.
- Initial goals of treatment are to restore nutritional status and address dehydration and electrolyte imbalance.
- Inpatient programs include supervised meals, weight monitoring, and psychoeducation.
- Pharmacological agents have not been shown to be effective in treating anorexia nervosa.
- Pharmacotherapy is used to treat comorbid illness such as depression.

BULIMIA NERVOSA

Epidemiology

- Bulimia nervosa affects 1 to 3 percent of young women and is more common in women.
- The age of onset is later in adolescence than with anorexia nervosa.

Etiology

- Patients with bulimia nervosa are highly influenced by societal pressure to be thin.
- They are also more likely to suffer from depression than the general population.
- They often feel neglected or rejected by their parents, and binge eating may satisfy feelings of deprivation.

Diagnostic criteria for Bulimia Nervosa

A. Recurrent episodes of binge eating. An episode of binge eating is characterized by both of the following:
   (1) eating, in a discrete period of time (e.g., within any 2-hour period), an amount of food that is definitely larger than most people would eat during a similar period of time and under similar circumstances
   (2) a sense of lack of control over eating during the episode (e.g., a feeling that one cannot stop eating or control what or how much one is eating)
B. Recurrent inappropriate compensatory behavior in order to prevent weight gain, such as self-induced vomiting; misuse of laxatives, diuretics, enemas, or other medications; fasting; or excessive exercise.
C. The binge eating and inappropriate compensatory behaviors both occur, on average, at least twice a week for 3 months.
D. Self-evaluation is unduly influenced by body shape and weight.
E. The disturbance does not occur exclusively during episodes of Anorexia Nervosa.

From American Psychiatric Association: Diagnostic and Statistical Manual of Mental Disorders, 4th ed., Text Revision. Washington, DC, American Psychiatric Association, 2000, with permission.

Course and Prognosis

- Bulimia nervosa has a chronic course that waxes and wanes over the long-term.
- The short-term outcome is variable but it is thought to have a better prognosis than anorexia nervosa.
- The prognosis depends on the extent of purging behavior and associated complications.
- Patients may develop electrolyte abnormalities, particularly hypomagnesemia and hyperamylasemia.
- Vomiting may also result in esophagitis, salivary gland enlargement, and dental erosion and caries.
- Patients can use ipecac to induce vomiting, and ipecac toxicity can result in cardiomyopathy.

Bulimia Nervosa (continued)

Treatment

- Patients with bulimia nervosa are not as secretive about their symptoms and are more agreeable to treatment than patients with anorexia nervosa.
- Treatment usually consists of a combination of psychotherapy and pharmacotherapy.
- Psychotherapy can occur in individual, group, and family settings.
- Bulimia nervosa may respond to antidepressant medication even in the absence of mood symptoms.

DIFFERENTIAL DIAGNOSIS

Anorexia Nervosa

Medical illness with anorexia (loss of appetite)
Depression associated with anorexia
Bulimia nervosa
Somatization disorder with weight fluctuation and vomiting
Schizophrenia with delusional thinking that revolves around food
Body dysmorphic disorder

Bulimia Nervosa

Depression associated with binge eating
Anorexia nervosa
Kluver-Bucy syndrome with compulsive licking and biting, hyperphagia, and hypersexuality
Kleine-Levin syndrome with 2–3 week periods of hypersomnia and hyperphagia
Borderline personality disorder with binge eating

Dementia: The Basics

IDENTIFICATION

There are 5 different dementias:

1) Dementia of the Alzheimer's Type

2) Vascular Dementia

3) Dementia Due to Other General Medical Conditions

4) Substance-Induced Persisting Dementia

5) Dementia Due to Multiple Etiologies

CHARACTERISTICS

Dementia is characterized by:
1) **memory impairment**
2) other **cognitive defects** such as impaired language abilities and decreased intellectual functioning
3) decline in social and occupational functioning

Dementia of the Alzheimer's Type is the most common type of dementia. It is characterized by memory impairment, at least one other symptom of cognitive decline, and deterioration in functioning.

Vascular Dementia is the second most common type of dementia. It is symptomatically similar to Alzheimer's, but includes focal neurological signs and clinical or laboratory evidence of a vascular etiology (e.g., a carotid bruit).

Dementia Due to Other General Medical Condition is a typical clinical picture of dementia. There are 6 specific medical conditions that are listed in the DSM-IV to cause dementia: (1) HIV infection, (2) head trauma, (3) Parkinson's disease, (4) Huntington's disease, (5) Pick's disease, and (6) Creutzfeldt-Jakob disease.

Substance-Induced Persisting Dementia is also the typical clinical picture of dementia. There are 5 specific substances that are listed in the DSM-IV to cause dementia: (1) alcohol, (2) inhalants, (3) sedatives, (4) hypnotics, and (5) anxiolytics.

Dementia Due to Multiple Etiologies is the clinical picture of dementia with evidence that the disturbance has more than one etiology (e.g., vascular and Alzheimer's together).

Dementia Not Otherwise Specified is a category used to diagnose dementia when the clinical picture is present, but the DSM-IV criteria are not met for any of the specific types.

Dementia: Essential Features

REVIEW

Dementia is mainly a disease of the elderly and it is estimated to affect 5 percent of people over 65 and 20 percent of people over 80. The hallmark of dementia is **memory impairment.** Dementia is also characterized by other **cognitive defects** and a **deterioration in social and occupational functioning.** Consciousness is *not* affected in dementia, and this is an important distinguishing factor between dementia and delirium, one of the main differentials. There are 5 different types of dementia but Alzheimer's type and vascular dementia together account for approximately 75 percent of all cases.

ESSENTIAL FEATURES

Alzheimer's type dementia

- Alzheimer's dementia is associated with genetic inheritance and a specific degeneration of **cholinergic** neurons.
- It affects the **cortex** with parietal-temporal atrophy, enlarged ventricles, and flattened sulci.
- **Amyloid plaques** and **neurofibrillary tangles** are present microscopically.
- There are impairments in memory, orientation, language, perception, and intellectual functioning.
- **Memory** for time and place is lost before memory for persons, and recent memory is lost before remote.
- **Orientation** can be affected and patients may not know how to return home from the grocery store or how to get back to the bedroom from the bathroom.
- **Language** may be vague, circumstantial, or stereotyped, and aphasia is a diagnostic criterion.
- **Perceptual** disturbances of hallucinations and delusions are present in 20 to 40 percent of patients.
- **Intellectual functioning** is impaired with poor concentration, and decreased problem-solving ability.
- **Personality changes** are common and patients may become angry, irritable, aggressive, sarcastic, or apathetic.
- **Depression** and **anxiety** can affect 40 to 50 percent of patients and mood lability may be apparent.
- Neurological signs such as **apraxia** and **agnosia** are also included in the diagnostic criteria.
- In **sundowner syndrome,** symptoms of dementia worsen in the evening, and it is characterized by drowsiness, confusion, ataxia, and accidental falls.
- Sundowner syndrome can occur in patients with dementia as a result of sedation with benzodiazepines or in the absence of external orienting cues such as light.
- Alzheimer's dementia is characterized by a **gradual decline** with **steady deterioration** in functioning.
- Patients with Alzheimer's type dementia survive an average of eight years from disease onset.
- It is treated with cholinesterase inhibitors for temporary improvement of cognitive function.
- Vitamin E and selegiline (Eldepryl) may slow disease progression.

Vascular Dementia

- Vascular dementia affects the **cortex** as a result of multiple cerebral infarctions.
- Infarctions are due to arteriosclerotic plaques or thromboemboli occluding the cerebral vessels.
- Vascular dementia is associated with hypertension or other risk factors of cardiovascular disease.
- Signs of vascular dementia include carotid bruits, funduscopic abnormalities, or cardiac valve disease.
- Vascular dementia appears clinically similar to Alzheimer's type with the classic impairments in **memory, orientation, language, perception,** and **intellectual functioning.**

Essential Features (continued)

- Vascular dementia is more likely to show neurological signs such as apraxia, aphasia, and agnosia.
- Personality changes are less common in vascular dementia as compared to Alzheimer's.
- Sundowner syndrome is also common in vascular dementia.
- Vascular dementia has a **sudden onset** of symptoms as each infarct causes abrupt impairment.
- The disease course is described as a **stepwise decline.**
- Vascular dementia is treated by reducing the risk factors associated with infarction (e.g., hypertension).

Alzheimer's type dementia	Vascular dementia
slow onset	abrupt onset
steady, gradual decline	stepwise decline with each infarct
personality changes are more prominent	focal neurological signs are more prominent
equal risk in men and women	men are at higher risk

HIV-Related Dementia
- HIV infection is associated with dementia at an annual rate of approximately 14 percent.
- HIV-related dementia does not include cases caused by opportunistic infections (e.g., cryptococcus).
- HIV primarily affects **subcortical** areas and the MMSE is ineffective for assessing dementia in these patients.

Head Trauma
- Head trauma occurs most commonly in young males.
- The dementia is a direct result of brain damage.
- The dementia is not progressive and cognitive deficit is stable over time.

Parkinson's Disease
- Twenty to 30 percent of patients with Parkinson's disease are estimated to have dementia.
- It is a disease of the basal ganglia with **Lewy bodies** and degeneration of the **substantia nigra.**
- The dementia is characterized by slowed thinking (*bradyphrenia*).

Huntington's Disease
- It is an autosomal dominant disease of the caudate nucleus with onset between 30 and 40 years old.
- Huntington's dementia is **subcortical** with more prominent motor abnormalities (choreoathetoid).
- Memory, language, and insight are likely to remain intact in early stages of the disease.
- Later stages are significant because of a high incidence of depression and psychosis.

Pick's Disease
- Pick's disease is characterized by atrophy in the frontal-temporal regions of the cortex.
- There are cytoskeletal elements called **Pick bodies** present.
- Personality and behavioral changes are predominant.

Creutzfeld-Jakob Disease
- Creutzfeld-Jakob disease is a rapidly progressive dementia with a prion as the infecting agent.
- The clinical triad is dementia, myoclonus, and EEG changes.
- A spongioform encephalopathy is present at autopsy.

Dementia: Depth and Detail

REVIEW

The most common types of dementia are Alzheimer's and vascular. There are also many other types of dementia associated with general medical conditions and substances. Each type of dementia may present with similar clinical symptoms, but certain characteristics vary according to the etiology. Approximately 15 percent of people with dementia may have reversible underlying pathology, so the attempt to elicit its cause is very important in diagnosing dementia. This section will review Alzheimer's type and vascular dementia in more detail.

ALZHEIMER'S TYPE DEMENTIA

Epidemiology
- Alzheimer's type is responsible for approximately 50 percent of all cases of dementia.
- Approximately forty percent of people with Alzheimer's have a family history of the disease.
- It is equally prevalent in men and women.

Etiology
- The cause of Alzheimer's disease is unknown.
- Among other genes, the apolipoprotein E4 (**apoE4**) gene has been implicated because its presence increases the chance of developing Alzheimer's.
- Neuropathological changes include amyloid protein deposition in the cortex (**senile plaques**), diffuse **cortical atrophy, neurofibrillary tangles,** and **cholinergic degeneration.**

Diagnostic criteria for Dementia of the Alzheimer's Type

A. The development of multiple cognitive deficits manifested by both
   (1) memory impairment (impaired ability to learn new information or to recall previously learned information)
   (2) one (or more) of the following cognitive disturbances:
      (a) aphasia (language disturbance)
      (b) apraxia (impaired ability to carry out motor activities despite intact motor function)
      (c) agnosia (failure to recognize or identify objects despite intact sensory function)
      (d) disturbance in executive functioning (i.e., planning, organizing, sequencing, abstracting)
B. The cognitive deficits in Criteria A1 and A2 each cause significant impairment in social or occupational functioning and represent a significant decline from a previous level of functioning.
C. The course is characterized by gradual onset and continuing cognitive decline.

Alzheimer's Type Dementia (continued)

D. The cognitive deficits in Criteria A1 and A2 are not due to any of the following:

    (1) other central nervous system conditions that cause progressive deficits in memory and cognition (e.g., cerebrovascular disease, Parkinson's disease, Huntington's disease, subdural hematoma, normal-pressure hydrocephalus, brain tumor)

    (2) systemic conditions that are known to cause dementia (e.g., hypthyroidism, vitamin B_{12} or folic acid deficiency, niacin deficiency, hypercalcemia, neurosyphilis, HIV infection)

    (3) substance-induced conditions

E. The deficits do not occur exclusively during the course of a delirium.

F. The disturbance is not better accounted for by another Axis I disorder (e.g., Major Depressive Disorder, Schizophrenia).

From American Psychiatric Association: Diagnostic and Statistical Manual of Mental Disorders, 4th ed., Text Revision. Washington, DC, American Psychiatric Association, 2000, with permission.

Course and Prognosis

- Alzheimer's disease shows a **gradual decline** in cognitive abilities and a **steady deterioration** of general functioning.
- It usually begins in the 6th or 7th decade and patients survive an average of approximately 8 years from disease onset.

Treatment

- Alzheimer's type is treated with appropriate medical care, emotional support, and pharmacotherapy.
- Tacrine (Cognex) and donezepil (Aricept) are cholinesterase inhibitors that may transiently improve cognitive function.
- Vitamin E (1000 mg/day) and selegeline (Eldepryl) are also used to slow disease progression.
- Antipsychotics with low anticholinergic side effects (e.g., olanzapine) are used to treat psychotic symptoms and severe agitation.

VASCULAR DEMENTIA

Epidemiology

- A vascular origin is responsible for 15 to 30 percent of all cases of dementia.
- Vascular dementia occurs more frequently in men.
- **Risk factors** include hypertension, obesity, hyperlipidemia, cardiac disease, diabetes, and smoking.

Etiology

- Vascular dementia is caused by occlusion of the cerebral vessels.
- Occlusion is the result of atherosclerotic plaques or thromboemboli.
- Vascular occlusion causes infarction and parenchymal lesions of the cortex.

Diagnostic criteria for Vascular Dementia

A. The development of multiple cognitive deficits manifested by both
    (1) memory impairment (impaired ability to learn new information or to recall previously learned information)
    (2) one (or more) of the following cognitive disturbances:
    (a) aphasia (language disturbance)
    (b) apraxia (impaired ability to carry out motor activities despite intact motor function)
    (c) agnosia (failure to recognize or identify objects despite intact sensory function)
    (d) disturbance in executive functioning (i.e., planning, organizing, sequencing, abstracting)
B. The cognitive deficits in Criteria A1 and A2 each cause significant impairment in social or occupational functioning and represent a significant decline from a previous level of functioning.
C. Focal neurological signs and symptoms (e.g., exaggeration of deep tendon reflexes, extensor plantar response, pseudobulbar palsy, gait abnormalities, weakness of an extremity) or laboratory evidence indicative of cerebrovascular disease (e.g., multiple infarctions involving cortex and underlying white matter) that are judged to be etiologically related to the disturbance.
D. The deficits do not occur exclusively during the course of a delirium.

From American Psychiatric Association: Diagnostic and Statistical Manual of Mental Disorders, 4th ed., Text Revision. Washington, DC, American Psychiatric Association, 2000, with permission.

Course and Prognosis
*   Vascular dementia has a **sudden onset** of symptoms and a **stepwise deterioration** in functioning.
*   The prognosis varies according to the severity of the vascular disease and control of the risk factors.

Treatment
*   The treatment is to reduce the risk factors associated with repeated infarcts.
*   Zolpidem is an effective medication for insomnia.
*   Antipsychotics may be used to treat perceptual disturbances such as delusions and hallucinations and severe agitation.

DIFFERENTIAL DIAGNOSIS

All causes of dementia: delirium, amnesia, depression, schizophrenia, and normal aging.

Delirium

- Delirium is characterized by cognitive impairments *and* a **change in consciousness** that develop over a short period of time.
- Delirium is caused by central nervous system disease, systemic disease, and substance intoxication or withdrawal.
- In the elderly, systemic infection is a likely cause (particularly urinary tract infection).
- Psychiatric symptoms of delirium include disturbance in mood, behavior, and perception.
- Neurological symptoms include urinary incontinence, tremor, asterixis, nystagmus, and ataxia.
- Symptoms may fluctuate over the course of a day with periods of complete lucidity.

Delirium	Dementia
sudden onset (hours to days)	gradual onset (weeks to years)
consciousness is decreased	consciousness is intact
cognitive impairments fluctuate	impairment is stable over time
a precipitant is usually identifiable	an identifiable precipitant is not required

Amnesia

- Amnesia is characterized by memory impairment alone *without* other cognitive defects.
- **Anterograde** amnesia is an impairment in the ability to learn **new** information.
- **Retrograde** amnesia is an impairment in the ability to recall **previously learned** information.
- Amnesia is caused by general medical conditions or drug use and a precipitant *must* be identified.
- Common medical causes include **head trauma, hypoxia, herpes encephalitis,** or **seizures.**
- **Alcohol** use is the most common substance-related cause of amnesia.
- Alcohol use may also lead to thiamine deficiency and Korsakoff syndrome with anterograde amnesia.
- Benzodiazepine use is also associated with amnesia (e.g., midazolam).

Depression

- Patients with depression may also have symptoms of cognitive impairment termed **pseudodementia.**
- These patients complain of memory impairment but actually suffer from depression.
- They are more likely to have a history of depression or a family history of psychiatric illness.
- The cognitive impairments subside if the depression is properly treated.

Pseudodementia	Dementia
abrupt onset	gradual onset
patients complain a lot of cognitive impairment	patients tend not to complain
specific complaints are detailed	complaints are vague
patients emphasize disability	patients conceal disability
patients appear highly distressed	patients do not appear too concerned
patients make little effort to perform tasks	patients struggle to perform
patients often give "I don't know" answers	near-miss answers are frequent
task performance is variable	task performance is consistently poor
remote and recent memory is impaired	remote memory is usually intact
dysfunction is worse upon waking	dysfunction is worse at night (sundowning)

Normal Aging

- A small degree of memory impairment can occur as a result of normal aging.
- Normal aging does *not* cause significant social or occupational deterioration.
- It is also referred to as benign senescent forgetfulness or age-associated memory impairment.

Somatoform Disorders: The Basics

IDENTIFICATION

There are 5 somatoform disorders:

1) Somatization Disorder

2) Conversion Disorder

3) Hypochondriasis

4) Body Dysmorphic Disorder

5) Pain Disorder

CHARACTERISTICS

The somatoform disorders are characterized by:
1) physical symptoms without medical cause
2) symptoms are *not* intentionally produced
3) psychological factors are associated with symptoms
4) persistent requests for medical attention

Somatization Disorder is characterized by a variety of physical complaints that include 4 pain symptoms, 2 gastrointestinal symptoms, 1 sexual symptom, and 1 neurological symptom other than pain.

Conversion Disorder is characterized by neurological symptoms that usually involve sensory or motor functioning such as functional blindness or paralysis.

Hypochondriasis is characterized by a preoccupation with the idea of having a serious disease.

Body Dysmorphic Disorder is characterized by a preoccupation with an imagined bodily defect.

Pain Disorder is characterized by physical complaints of pain that require medical attention but have a psychological origin.

Somatoform Disorders: Essential Features

REVIEW

Somatoform disorders are characterized by persistent requests for medical attention because of physical complaints that cannot be sufficiently explained by medical causes. The symptoms are associated with psychological stressors but are *not* intentionally produced. Somatoform disorders probably occur through some mechanism that allows unconscious conflict to manifest as physical symptoms. The nature of the mechanism is not fully understood and may vary according to the specific somatoform disorder. The following section will review the essential features of the somatoform disorders.

ESSENTIAL FEATURES

Somatization Disorder
- Four pain, 2 gastrointestinal, 1 sexual, and 1 neurological symptom are required for diagnosis.
- **Pain** occurs in sites such as the abdomen, head, back, and extremities.
- **Gastrointestinal symptoms** are usually nausea and vomiting.
- The **sexual symptom** can be related to menstruation or sexual functioning, but *cannot* include pain.
- Examples of **neurological symptoms** are paralysis or weakness, but *not* pain.
- Somatization disorder is associated with anxiety, depression, and cluster B personality disorders (especially histrionic PD).
- The disease usually begins in adolescence, and patients suffer a chronic debilitating course.
- Patients with somatization disorder frequently threaten suicide, but rarely make attempts.
- Complaints should be addressed as emotional, *not* medical.
- Treatment is with psychotherapy.

Conversion Disorder
- Conversion disorder is characterized by motor and neurological symptoms.
- The most common neurological symptoms are paralysis, blindness, and mutism.
- Motor symptoms include weakness, impaired balance, and abnormal movements.
- **Pseudoseizures** are a common symptom in conversion disorder.
- **La belle indifference** is characteristic of conversion disorder, in which patients are not appropriately concerned about what appear to be serious symptoms.
- It is frequently associated with anxiety, depression, and cluster B personality disorders.
- Symptoms usually remit spontaneously within days but approximately 25 percent of patients may experience relapses.

Hypochondriasis
- Hypochondriasis is characterized by a persistent fear of contracting, or having, a serious medical illness.
- It is thought to result from the inaccurate interpretation of physical symptoms.
- Symptoms must occur for at least **6 months** and convince patients they have a particular disease.
- There is no evidence to support the presence of a disease, but still patients cannot be dissuaded.
- Transient hypochondriacal states may exist following true illness or the death of a loved one.
- Hypochondriasis is associated with psychiatric symptoms of anxiety and depression.
- It follows a chronic waxing and waning course with symptom exacerbation during stressful times.
- Reassurance through psychotherapy and regular physical exams may be helpful.

Essential Features (continued)

Body Dysmorphic Disorder

- Patients with body dysmorphic disorder are preoccupied with an imagined or grossly exaggerated bodily defect.
- The distress may be so severe that patients refuse to leave the house for fear of being ridiculed.
- The most common perceived defects involve facial structure, such as a deformed nose.
- Affected body parts may change throughout the course of the disorder.
- **Ideas of reference** (people supposedly noticing the flaw), **compulsive checking** of the defect, or **rituals** to cover it up often accompany the disorder.
- It is also associated with social phobia, obsessive-compulsive disorder, and major depression.
- The disorder typically follows a chronic, debilitating course.
- Antidepressants may reduce symptoms in the majority of patients.

Pain Disorder

- Pain in general is the most common reason to seek medical attention.
- The main presenting complaint is pain that cannot be *fully* explained by a medical condition.
- In order to diagnosis pain disorder, the pain may be partially caused by a medical condition (e.g., status post trauma) but must also have psychological factors associated with it.
- The pain may affect any part of the body.
- Patients usually have long medical histories and often insist on treatment with medication or surgery.
- Patients blame the pain as the source of all their distress and deny any emotional component.
- They may self-medicate by using drugs and/or alcohol.
- Depressive symptoms are extremely common in pain disorder.
- Patients may suffer a chronic course and prognosis depends on the underlying psychological factors.
- Amitriptyline (Elavil) has been shown to be effective in treating chronic pain.

Somatoform Disorders: Depth and Detail

REVIEW

Hypochondriasis and pain disorder are the only somatoform disorders that occur with any regular frequency in the general population. Hypochondriasis is also the only somatoform disorder that affects men and women equally, the rest are more prevalent in women. Genetic influences play an etiological role in these disorders, but issues of primary and secondary gain also clearly contribute to their development. In **primary gain,** patients develop physical symptoms in an unconscious effort to keep intrapsychic conflict outside of their awareness. In **secondary gain,** patients derive specific benefits from the physical symptoms (e.g., avoiding obligations, emotional support). Somatoform disorders tend to follow a chronic course, and management is achieved through psychotherapy and pharmacotherapy. This section will review important details of somatoform disorders and discuss the differential diagnosis.

SOMATIZATION DISORDER

Epidemiology
- Somatization disorder occurs in less than 1 percent of the general population.
- It is more common in women and people with low socioeconomic status.

Etiology
- Biological theories suggest that these patients may not accurately interpret somatosensory input.
- Somatic complaints may also allow the patient to avoid obligations (secondary gain).

Diagnostic criteria for Somatization Disorder

A. A history of many physical complaints beginning before age 30 years that occur over a period of several years and result in treatment being sought or significant impairment in social, occupational, or other important areas of functioning.

B. Each of the following criteria must have been met, with individual symptoms occurring at any time during the course of the disturbance:

   (1) *four pain symptoms:* a history of pain related to at least four different sites or functions (e.g., head, abdomen, back, joints, extremities, chest, rectum, during menstruation, during sexual intercourse, or during urination)

   (2) *two gastrointestinal symptoms:* a history of at least two gastrointestinal symptoms other than pain (e.g., nausea, bloating, vomiting other than during pregnancy, diarrhea, or intolerance of several different foods)

   (3) *one sexual symptom:* a history of at least one sexual or reproductive symptom other than pain (e.g., sexual indifference, erectile or ejaculatory dysfunction, irregular menses, excessive menstrual bleeding, vomiting throughout pregnancy)

   (4) *one pseudoneurological symptom:* a history of at least one symptom or deficit suggesting a neurological condition not limited to pain (conversion symptoms such as impaired coordination or balance, paralysis or localized weakness, difficulty swallowing or lump in throat, aphonia, urinary retention, hallucinations, loss of touch or pain sensation, double vision, blindness, deafness, seizures; dissociative symptoms such as amnesia; or loss of consciousness other than fainting)

Somatization Disorder (continued)

C. Either (1) or (2):

(1) after appropriate investigation, each of the symptoms in Criterion B cannot be fully explained by a known general medical condition or the direct effects of a substance (e.g., a drug abuse, a medication)

(2) when there is a related general medical condition, the physical complaints or resulting social or occupational impairment are in excess of what would be expected from the history, physical examination, or laboratory findings.

D. The symptoms are not intentionally produced or feigned (as in Factitious Disorder or Malingering)

From American Psychiatric Association: Diagnostic and Statistical Manual of Mental Disorders, 4th ed., Text Revision. Washington, DC, American Psychiatric Association, 2000, with permission.

Course and Prognosis
- The disorder usually begins during adolescence and it must begin before age 30 for diagnosis.
- It is usually chronic and debilitating with symptom exacerbation associated with psychological stressors.

Treatment
- Somatic complaints should be treated as emotional rather than medical.
- Psychotherapy is useful to help the patient appreciate the psychological component of the disorder.
- Comorbid depression or anxiety should be treated with medication.

CONVERSION DISORDER

Epidemiology
- The prevalence of conversion disorder varies according to the population.
- It is more common in women and people with low socioeconomic status.

Etiology
- Psychoanalytic theory views conversion disorder as the result of repressed intrapsychic conflicts.
- The anxiety that unconscious conflicts cause is *converted* into physical symptoms.
- Brain-imaging studies indicate that biological factors may also contribute to conversion disorder.

Diagnostic criteria for Conversion Disorder

A. One or more symptoms or deficits affecting voluntary motor or sensory function that suggest a neurological or other general medical condition.

B. Psychological factors are judged to be associated with the symptom or deficit because the initiation or exacerbation of the symptom or deficit is preceded by conflicts or other stressors.

C. The symptom or deficit is not intentionally produced or feigned (as in Factitious Disorder or Malingering).

D. The symptom or deficit cannot, after appropriate investigation, be fully explained by a general medical condition, or by the direct effects of a substance, or as a culturally sanctioned behavior or experience.

E. The symptom or deficit causes clinically significant distress or impairment in social, occupational, or other important areas of functioning or warrants medical evaluation.

F. The symptom or deficit is not limited to pain or sexual dysfunction, does not occur exclusively during the course of Somatization Disorder, and is not better accounted for by another mental disorder.

From American Psychiatric Association: Diagnostic and Statistical Manual of Mental Disorders, 4th ed., Text Revision. Washington, DC, American Psychiatric Association, 2000, with permission.

Conversion Disorder (continued)

Course and Prognosis

- Initial symptoms usually resolve within a few days and many patients will not have another episode.
- Approximately 25 percent of patients will have additional episodes associated with stress.
- A good prognosis is associated with short symptomatic periods and identifiable precipitating factors.

Treatment

- Recovery may be spontaneous.
- Cognitive-behavioral therapy and psychoanalytic psychotherapy have been shown to be helpful.
- Hypnosis, relaxation training, and biofeedback techniques may also be effective.
- Pharmacotherapy is used to treat comorbid depression and anxiety.

HYPOCHONDRIASIS

Epidemiology

- Hypochondriasis affects approximately 5 percent of people who seek medical attention.
- It is equally prevalent in men and women, and socioeconomic status is *not* a factor.

Etiology

- Patients may have a lower tolerance for physical pain.
- They may be unknowingly looking to enter the sick role and avoid obligations (secondary gain).
- Hypochondriasis could also be a manifestation of an underlying depressive or anxiety disorder.

Diagnostic criteria for Hypochondriasis

A. Preoccupation with fears of having, or the idea that one has, a serious disease based on the person's misinterpretation of bodily symptoms.

B. The preoccupation persists despite appropriate medical evaluation and reassurance.

C. The belief in Criterion A is not of delusional intensity (as in Delusional Disorder, Somatic Type) and is not restricted to a circumscribed concern about appearance (as in Body Dysmorphic Disorder).

D. The preoccupation causes clinically significant distress or impairment in social, occupational, or other important areas of functioning.

E. The duration of the disturbance is at least 6 months.

F. The preoccupation is not better accounted for by Generalized Anxiety Disorder, Obsessive-Compulsive Disorder, Panic Disorder, a Major Depressive Episode, Separation Anxiety, or another Somatoform Disorder.

From American Psychiatric Association: Diagnostic and Statistical Manual of Mental Disorders, 4th ed., Text Revision. Washington, DC, American Psychiatric Association, 2000, with permission.

Course and Prognosis

- Hypochondriasis usually has episodes that last months to years with asymptomatic periods in between.
- There are often obvious psychological stressors associated with symptom exacerbation.
- Up to 50 percent of patients show significant improvement.

Hypochondriasis (continued)

Treatment
- Psychotherapy in a group setting may be effective.
- Regular physical exams may serve to reassure patients.
- Pharmacotherapy is currently used only to treat comorbid depressive and anxiety disorders, but several SSRI trials are underway.

BODY DYSMORPHIC DISORDER

Epidemiology
- The prevalence of body dysmorphic disorder is unknown.
- It is more likely to occur in women, and the most common age of onset is between 15 and 20.

Etiology
- The pathophysiology of body dysmorphic disorder may be related to serotonin dysregulation.
- Patients are more likely to have a family history of depression or obsessive-compulsive disorder.
- Cultural concepts of beauty also impact patients with this disorder.

Diagnostic criteria for Body Dysmorphic Disorder

A. Preoccupation with an imagined defect in appearance. If a slight physical anomaly is present, the person's concern is markedly excessive.
B. The preoccupation causes clinically significant distress or impairment in social, occupational, or other important areas of functioning.
C. The preoccupation is not better accounted for by another mental disorder (e.g., dissatisfaction with body shape and size in Anorexia Nervosa).

From American Psychiatric Association: Diagnostic and Statistical Manual of Mental Disorders, 4th ed., Text Revision. Washington, DC, American Psychiatric Association, 2000, with permission.

Course and Prognosis
- Disease onset is gradual.
- Patients become progressively distressed about the perceived defect until functioning is impaired.
- A chronic waxing and waning disease course is characteristic.
- As symptoms of one preoccupation remit, the patient may focus on a new perceived defect.

Treatment
- Initial treatment is often mistakenly focused on cosmetic repair (e.g., dental, surgical, or dermatological).
- Serotonin reuptake inhibitors will reduce symptoms in a majority of patients.

PAIN DISORDER

Epidemiology

- Pain (lower back pain in particular) is the most common reason for a person to seek medical attention.
- Pain disorder is more common in women and usually occurs between age 30 and 50.

Etiology

- Pain disorder is thought to be an expression of unconscious conflicts.
- It may be an unconscious method to achieve secondary gain.
- Biological factors include a hypothesized endorphin deficiency.
- Psychogenic causes are likely when the pain does not vary in intensity or respond to analgesics.

Diagnostic Criteria for Pain Disorder

A. Pain in one or more anatomical sites is the predominant focus of the clinical presentation and is of sufficient severity to warrant clinical attention.
B. The pain causes clinically significant distress or impairment in social, occupational, or other important areas of functioning.
C. Psychological factors are judged to have an important role in the onset, severity, exacerbation, or maintenance of the pain.
D. The symptom or deficit is not intentionally produced or feigned (as in Factitious Disorder or Malingering).
E. The pain is not better accounted for by a Mood, Anxiety, or Psychotic Disorder and does not meet criteria for Dyspareunia.

From American Psychiatric Association: Diagnostic and Statistical Manual of Mental Disorders, 4th ed., Text Revision. Washington, DC, American Psychiatric Association, 2000, with permission.

Course and Prognosis

- The onset of the disorder is usually sudden.
- It may become progressively worse and result in chronic debilitation.
- Prognosis varies, and depends on the underlying psychological factors.

Treatment

- It may not be possible to reduce the pain, and analgesics are rarely effective.
- Psychotherapy is used to address the underlying psychological factors.
- Biofeedback training and relaxation techniques may be effective.
- Antidepressant medications such as amitriptyline (Elavil) are useful for unclear reasons.

DIFFERENTIAL DIAGNOSIS

Medical

Brain tumors

Myasthenia gravis

Multiple sclerosis

Systemic lupus eythematosus

Polymyositis

Guillain-Barré syndrome

AIDS

Psychiatric (may present with somatic complaints)

Schizophrenia

Depressive disorders

Anxiety disorders

Personality disorders

Malingering

- Malingering is an *intentional* production of false or exaggerated physical or psychological symptoms.
- Symptom production is motivated by **external incentives.**
- Examples of external incentives are: (1) avoiding military duty, (2) avoiding work, (3) financial compensation, (4) evading criminal prosecution, and (5) obtaining drugs.
- The symptoms of malingering are usually reported in a vague or overly dramatized manner.
- Symptoms are not consistent with known clinical conditions.
- Findings may appear consistent with self-inflicted injury.
- History may reveal past episodes of injury or undiagnosed illness.
- There is often a marked discrepancy between claimed disability and objective findings.
- Malingerers are rarely cooperative with the evaluation or treatment.
- Antisocial personality traits or personality disorder is a common comorbid finding.
- Suspect malingering whenever patients are referred by an attorney (secondary gain).

Factitious Disorder

- In factitious disorder the patient *intentionally* produces symptoms in order to enter the sick role.
- External incentives are absent (as opposed to malingering).
- Another name for factitious disorder is Munchausen syndrome
- These patients may demonstrate psychiatric *or* physical symptoms.
- Feigned psychiatric symptoms include depression, hallucinations, and bizarre behavior.
- Physical symptoms such as hypoglycemia are produced by injecting insulin, bleeding is induced by taking anti-coagulants, or hyperthyroidism can be simulated by taking thyroid hormone.
- These patients are very knowledgeable about the disease they are trying to produce.
- They usually have a long medical history from many hospitals and it may include multiple surgeries.
- Factitious disorder by proxy may also occur where symptoms are intentionally produced in *another* person who is under the perpetrator's care.
- In factitious disorder by proxy the perpetrator is able to indirectly assume the sick role.

Dissociative Disorders: The Basics

IDENTIFICATION

There are 4 dissociative disorders:

1) Dissociative Amnesia

2) Dissociative Fugue

3) Dissociative Identity Disorder

4) Depersonalization Disorder

CHARACTERISTICS

Dissociative disorders are characterized by:
1) identity disturbance
2) memory disturbance
3) perceptual disturbance (e.g., depersonalization and derealization)

Dissociative amnesia is the inability to recall certain traumatic or distressing events.

Dissociative fugue occurs when a patient unexpectedly travels away from home and is unable to recall their identity.

Dissociative identity disorder is characterized by the presence of 2 or more distinct identity states that control the patient's behavior at different times.

Depersonalization Disorder is described as the feeling of detachment from various aspects of the self. Reality testing remains intact but patients report a feeling of being "outside" of their bodies and feeling detached from their sense of self.

Dissociative Disorders: Essential Features

REVIEW

Dissociation is usually the result of trauma. The patient is unable to cope with the psychological ramifications of the trauma, and dissociation is the process that removes it from consciousness. Dissociation may also occur suddenly during the trauma to allow the person to withstand the actual incident. Dissociation has traditionally been considered a defense mechanism but it is now clear that there are also biological underpinnings. This section will review the essential features of the dissociative disorders.

ESSENTIAL FEATURES

Dissociative Amnesia
- Amnesia is the most common dissociative symptom.
- Dissociative amnesia usually has an abrupt onset and the patient *is aware* of the memory loss.
- It occurs in response to a painful or stressful event that the patient has trouble handling.
- Such events may include natural disasters, witnessing violence, accidents, or abuse.
- There are several different forms of dissociative amnesia that refer to the period of forgotten time.
- *Localized* amnesia is the most common, where memory for a specific period of time is lost (hrs-days).
- *Selective* amnesia is the loss of memory for some events, but not *all* the events in a specific period.
- In *generalized* amnesia, memories across an entire lifetime cannot be recalled.
- Amnesia is often associated with primary and secondary gain.
- Depression and anxiety frequently co-exist with dissociative amnesia.
- The symptoms of dissociative amnesia usually end abruptly.
- Barbiturates and benzodiazepines may be useful in recovering lost memories.

Dissociative Fugue
- Patients in a fugue state usually wander far away from home for several hours or days.
- During the fugue patients may assume another identity and always lose their prior identity.
- Unlike dissociative amnesia, patients in a fugue state *do not realize* that they have forgotten anything.
- They tend not to exhibit strange or unusual behavior during the fugue.
- Fugue periods are brief, and memory for personal information and identity may return suddenly.
- After recovery, patients remain amnestic for the fugue period itself.

Essential Features (continued)

Dissociative Identity Disorder

- Dissociative identity disorder was previously called multiple personality disorder.
- Patients have at least 2 identities and may switch rapidly from one to another.
- Identity is defined as discrete self-states with their own characteristics and ability to dictate consciousness and executive function.
- They may or may not be aware that other identities exist.
- Identities may be of any gender, age, or species.
- Different personality types may also exist in which one is talkative and extroverted and the other is shy.
- Patients may report time lapses and memory loss for the times when different identities are dominant.
- They sometimes use the pronoun "we" to refer to themselves.
- A history of severe emotional, physical, or sexual abuse as a young child is common.
- Patients report that voices are coming from within themselves rather than from outside, or separate.
- The mental status exam may not reveal anything characteristic except for periods of amnesia.
- Patients may initially appear to have borderline personality disorder or schizophrenia.
- The disease tends to run a chronic course with recovery presenting a serious clinical challenge.
- Insight-oriented psychodynamic psychotherapy is the treatment of choice.

Depersonaliztion Disorder

- The symptom of depersonalization may occur as a transient phenomenon that is *not* pathological.
- Patients with depersonalization disorder feel like they are detached from various aspects of the self such as body, thoughts, feelings, and movements.
- These patients feel strange and unreal, like they exist in a dream.
- A doubling phenomenon may occur where patients feel like they are observing themselves from a distance rather than fully participating in their actions.
- Patients recognize these symptoms as abnormal, or ego-dystonic (unacceptable to the self).
- Patients may suffer a chronic unremitting course or waxing and waning symptom exacerbation.
- There is no treatment modality that is currently recommended.

Dissociative Disorders: Depth and Detail

REVIEW

The dissociative disorders are uncommon. Dissociative states are usually the result of psychological stressors and their treatment revolves around identifying those stressors. Dissociative disorders such as fugue and amnesia frequently resolve abruptly without significant sequelae. This section will review the important details of dissociative disorders and include a differential diagnosis.

DISSOCIATIVE AMNESIA

Epidemiology
- Amnesia is the most common dissociative symptom and it occurs in most dissociative disorders.
- Dissociative amnesia is more frequently seen in female adolescents and young adults.

Etiology
- Memory recall is affected by the emotional content of the amnestic events, where memories the patient cannot recall are usually traumatic and stressful.
- Dissociation is considered a combination of biological process *and* psychological defense mechanism.

Diagnostic criteria for Dissociative Amnesia

A. The predominant disturbance is one or more episodes of inability to recall important personal information, usually of a traumatic or stressful nature, that is too extensive to be explained by ordinary forgetfulness.
B. The disturbance does not occur exclusively during the course of Dissociative Identity Disorder, Dissociative Fugue, Posttraumatic Stress Disorder, Acute Stress Disorder, or Somatization Disorder and is not due to the direct physiological effects of a substance (e.g., a drug of abuse, a medication) or a neurological or other general medical condition (e.g., Amnestic Disorder Due to Head Trauma).
C. The symptoms cause clinically significant distress or impairment in social, occupational, or other important areas of functioning.

From American Psychiatric Association: Diagnostic and Statistical Manual of Mental Disorders, 4th ed., Text Revision. Washington, DC, American Psychiatric Association, 2000, with permission.

Course and Prognosis
- The symptoms of dissociative amnesia usually begin and end suddenly.
- Patients may experience recurrences, but recovery is usually complete.
- Prognosis depends on how easily memories can be restored.

Treatment
- Barbiturates and benzodiazepines are useful in recovering lost memories.
- Hypnosis and relaxation techniques may facilitate recall.
- Follow-up with psychotherapy is recommended to ensure recovery.

DISSOCIATIVE FUGUE

Epidemiology
- Dissociative fugue is very rare.

Etiology
- Patients are *psychologically* motivated to withdraw from emotionally painful experiences.
- Common stressors include marital, financial, and occupational difficulties.

Diagnostic criteria for Dissociative Fugue

A. The predominant disturbance is sudden, unexpected travel away from home or one's customary place of work, with inability to recall one's past.
B. Confusion about personal identity or assumption of a new identity (partial or complete).
C. The disturbance does not occur exclusively during the course of Dissociative Identity Disorder and is not due to the direct physiological effects of a substance (e.g., a drug of abuse, a medication) or a general medical condition (e.g., temporal lobe epilepsy).
D. The symptoms cause clinically significant distress or impairment in social, occupational, or other important areas of functioning.

From American Psychiatric Association: Diagnostic and Statistical Manual of Mental Disorder, 4th ed., Text Revision. Washington, DC, American Psychiatric Association, 2000, with permission.

Course and Prognosis
- Fugue periods are usually brief, lasting hours to days.
- Recovery is spontaneous and recurrences generally do not occur.

Treatment
- Barbiturates, benzodiazepines, hypnosis, and relaxation techniques all may be useful to facilitate recall.
- Psychotherapy follow-up is recommended.

DISSOCIATIVE IDENTITY DISORDER

Epidemiology
- Estimates of the prevalence of dissociative identity disorder vary widely.
- The disorder is most common in adolescents and overwhelmingly diagnosed in women.
- It can also develop in young children.

Etiology
- Severe childhood sexual or physical abuse is usually the causative factor.
- Other proposed factors include other traumatic events and a genetic predisposition.
- There is evidence that the disorder is more common in first-degree biological relatives.

Dissociative Identity Disorder (continued)

Diagnostic criteria for Dissociative Identity Disorder

A. The presence of two or more distinct identities or personality states (each with its own relatively enduring pattern of perceiving, relating to, and thinking about the environment and self).

B. At least two of these identities or personality states recurrently take control of the person's behavior.

C. Inability to recall important personal information that is too extensive to be explained by ordinary forgetfulness.

D. The disturbance is not due to the direct physiological effects of a substance (e.g., blackouts or chaotic behavior during Alcohol Intoxication) or a general medical condition (e.g., complex partial seizures).   **Note:** In children, the symptoms are not attributable to imaginary playmates or other fantasy play.

From American Psychiatric Association: Diagnostic and Statistical Manual of Mental Disorders, 4th ed., Text Revision. Washington, DC, American Psychiatric Association, 2000, with permission.

Course and Prognosis

- Female adolescents are most frequently affected and have been noted to follow 2 symptom patterns.
- One pattern is of sexual promiscuity, drug use, somatic symptoms, and suicide attempts.
- Another pattern is characterized by social withdrawal and childlike behavior.
- Prognosis is related to age of onset where the earlier the onset, the worse the prognosis.
- Dissociative identity disorder is the most severe and chronic of the dissociative disorders.
- Recovery is difficult and usually incomplete.

Treatment

- Insight-oriented psychodynamic psychotherapy is the most effective approach to this disorder.
- Hypnosis and barbiturates may be used to facilitate disclosure during interviews.
- Antidepressants and anxiolytics may be useful to treat associated psychiatric symptoms.
- Hospitalization may be required for suicidal or impulsive behavior.

DEPERSONALIZATION DISORDER

Epidemiology

- Prevalence rates of depersonalization disorder are unknown.
- Depersonalization may occur as a transient phenomenon that is *not* pathological.
- Depersonalization is often a symptom of depression, anxiety, and schizophrenia.

Etiology

- Psychological factors such as severe stress can play a role in depersonalization disorder.
- Neurological disorders such as temporal lobe epilepsy and brain tumors have been associated.
- Systemic disease or substance abuse may also cause depersonalization symptoms.

Diagnostic criteria for Depersonalization Disorder

A. Persistent or recurrent experiences of feeling detached from, and as if one is an outside observer of, one's mental processes or body (e.g., feeling like one is in a dream).

B. During the depersonalization experience, reality testing remains intact.

C. The depersonalization causes clinically significant distress or impairment in social, occupational, or other important areas of functioning.

D. The depersonalization experience does not occur exclusively during the course of another mental disorder, such as Schizophrenia, Panic Disorder, Acute Stress Disorder, or another Dissociative Disorder, and is not due to the direct physiological effects of a substance (e.g., a drug of abuse, a medication) or a general medical condition (e.g., temporal lobe epilepsy).

From American Psychiatric Association: Diagnostic and Statistical Manual of Mental Disorders, 4th ed., Text Revision. Washington, DC, American Psychiatric Association, 2000, with permission.

Course and Prognosis

- Symptoms usually first appear abruptly and onset is between 15 and 30 years old.
- The disorder may follow a chronic unremitting course for many patients.
- Other patients experience periodic symptom exacerbation that varies in severity.
- Anxiety (e.g., panic attacks) can trigger the onset of symptoms.

Treatment

- Specific treatment regimens have not been investigated in depersonalization disorder.
- Comorbid psychiatric illness should be treated accordingly.

DIFFERENTIAL DIAGNOSIS

Medical

Dementia

Delirium

Anoxia

Cerebral infection

Brain tumors

Substance-induced (alcohol, hypnotics, anticholinergics, steroids, PCP, marijuana, and hallucinogens)

Temporal lobe epilepsy

Head trauma

Transient global amnesia

Wernicke-Korsakoff syndrome

Psychiatric

Posttraumatic stress disorder

Acute stress disorder

Somatoform disorders

Malingering

Factitious disorder

Sleepwalking disorder

Psychotic disorders

Pseudologia fantastica (falsification of memory)

Ganser's Syndrome

- Ganser's syndrome is classified as a dissociative disorder not otherwise specified (NOS).
- It is usually considered a variant of malingering.
- It is generally associated with prison inmates who want to avoid punishment.
- Ganser's syndrome is the *intentional* production of *psychiatric* symptoms.
- The syndrome is characterized by giving approximate answers to specific questions.
- People with this disorder respond with near-correct answers such as 2 plus 2 equals 5.
- Symptoms usually do not resemble any known diagnostic entity.
- Patients display exacerbations of symptoms when they are being watched.
- Recovery is sudden and patients typically claim to have amnesia for the symptomatic episode.

Sleep Disorders: The Basics

IDENTIFICATION

1) Insomnia

2) Narcolepsy

3) Obstructive Sleep Apnea

4) Circadian Rhythm Disorder

5) Nightmare Disorder

6) Sleep Terror Disorder

7) Sleepwalking Disorder

CHARACTERISTICS

Sleep disorders are characterized by disturbances in the sleep/wake cycle:

Insomnia is a difficulty in falling asleep or staying asleep in which patients do not feel fully rested.

Narcolepsy is characterized by increased REM sleep, hypersomnia, and episodes of "sleep attacks."

Obstructive Sleep Apnea is characterized by multiple episodes of absent airflow during sleep.

Circadian Rhythm Disorder occurs when external sleep periods do not coincide with biological clocks.

Nightmare Disorder is characterized by frightening dreams that occur during **REM.**

Sleep Terror Disorder is characterized by waking up in a panic-like state during **non-REM sleep.**

Sleepwalking Disorder is leaving the bed and walking during stage 3 and 4 sleep (**non-REM**).

Sleep Disorders: Essential Features

REVIEW

The prevalence of sleep disorders is frequently underestimated and patients often resist seeking treatment. Sleep disorders may occur as a primary disturbance or secondary to underlying medical or psychiatric conditions. The importance of proper sleep should not be overlooked because of its relevance to health and daily functioning. This section will review the essential features of the primary sleep disorders.

ESSENTIAL FEATURES

Insomnia

- Insomnia is the most common sleep complaint.
- It may be chronic or occur transiently in response to discomfort or environmental stress.
- There are 3 kinds of insomnia: (1) difficulty falling asleep, (2) difficulty staying asleep, and (3) early morning wakening.
- **Difficulty falling asleep** is usually associated with **anxiety.**
- **Multiple awakenings** throughout the course of the night may indicate **organic disease.**
- **Waking up early** in the morning is usually associated with **depression.**
- Patients who complain of insomnia tend to overestimate the extent of sleep deprivation.
- Daily functioning is affected because of decreased concentration, decreased energy, and irritability.
- Insomnia is treated by improving sleep hygiene and administering sedative/hypnotic medication.

Narcolepsy

- Narcolepsy is characterized by hypersomnia, sleep attacks, hypnagogic hallucinations, hypnopompic hallucinations, cataplexy, and sleep paralysis.
- **Hypersomnia** is defined as excessive daytime sleepiness.
- **Sleep attacks** may occur at any time and are the most common symptom of narcolepsy.
- **Hypnagogic hallucinations** are auditory or visual disturbances that occur **prior** to falling asleep.
- **Hynopompic hallucinations** are disturbances that occur **upon wakening.**
- **Cataplexy** is a sudden loss of muscle tone commonly associated with sleep attacks.
- **Sleep paralysis** occurs upon waking, in which patients are awake but unable to move for brief periods.
- REM sleep is also prolonged in narcolepsy and it first begins very early after sleep onset.
- REM sleep *normally* appears approximately 90 minutes after sleep onset, but in narcolepsy it begins after 10 minutes.
- Narcolepsy is treated with CNS stimulants such as pemoline (Cylert) and methylphenidate (Ritalin).

Obstructive Sleep Apnea (OSA)

- In OSA patients awake in the middle of the night gasping for air.
- The structural anatomy of the oropharynx predisposes these patients to obstructed airflow.
- An apneic event is defined as the cessation of airflow for 10 seconds or more.
- At least 30 apneic events per night are required for the diagnosis of OSA.
- Events usually occur during stage 3, 4, and REM sleep while pharyngeal muscles are more relaxed.
- Micro-awakenings deprive patients of deep sleep and cause **excessive daytime sleepiness.**
- OSA is frequently associated with **obesity** and **snoring.**
- OSA is usually treated with continuous positive airway pressure (CPAP) during sleep.

Essential Features (continued)

Circadian Rhythm Disorder

- In circadian rhythm disorder the patient's internal clock is not aligned with external sleep periods.
- Jet-lag is an example of a rhythm disorder where a traveler can feel like it is midnight at 7:00 AM.
- Circadian rhythm disorder also occurs in response to shift work (e.g., night float) or sleep phase delay.
- Sleep phase delay is characterized by a forward shift in sleep onset *and* wake times and is common in college students.
- Treatments vary according to the type of disturbance (e.g., melatonin for jet-lag)

Sleep Terror Disorder

- Sleep terrors are awakenings during stage 3 and 4 (non-REM) sleep in the first third of the night.
- They are more common in children, particularly boys.
- Patients may wake up screaming with feelings of anxiety or panic.
- They appear confused and disoriented upon awakening from a sleep terror.
- Unlike nightmare disorder, sleep terrors are usually of an image and not of a dream.
- They tend to fall back asleep afterward and forget that the episode occurred.
- Sleep terrors usually resolve spontaneously, but severe cases may be treated with benzodiazepines.

Nightmare Disorder

- Nightmares are frightening **dreams** that occur during REM sleep and awaken the patient.
- They typically occur in children in response to stressful life events or anxiety.
- Upon awakening, patients quickly become alert and oriented.
- There are no harmful effects of waking a patient in the midst of a nightmare.
- Nightmare disorders are usually self-limited.

Sleepwalking Disorder

- Sleepwalking occurs during stage 3 and 4 (non-REM) sleep in the first third of the night.
- It is more frequently seen in children and adolescents.
- Patients may perform complex motor movements such as dressing, walking, or even driving.
- Although patients may appear awake, communication is not possible.
- They usually return to bed without any memory of the event.
- The treatment is to wake the patient from sleepwalking to avert any risk of harm.

Sleep Disorders: Depth and Detail

REVIEW

This section will review the important details of the primary sleep disorders.

INSOMNIA

Epidemiology

- Insomnia is very common, and one-third of the population may suffer at some point in their lifetime.

Etiology

- It may be the result of stress and anxiety, depression, pain, or organic illness.

Diagnosis

- Sleep disorders are diagnosed with nighttime polysomnography (NPSG).
- Multiple sleep latency tests (MSLT) are administered in the afternoon and measure daytime sleepiness.

Course and Prognosis

- Patients with insomnia often do not seek treatment until functioning is severely impaired.
- Insomnia may be chronic or transient and related to environmental stressors.

Treatment

- Insomnia is treated with benzodiazepines, zolpidem, trazodone, or other sedative/hypnotics.
- Methods to improve sleep hygiene are effective in treating insomnia and include (1) arising at the same time each day, (2) using the bed only to sleep, (3) avoiding daytime naps, and (4) avoiding meals near bedtime.

NARCOLEPSY

Epidemiology

- Narcolepsy has a prevalence of less than 1 percent in the general population.
- The onset of narcolepsy is usually before age 30 and it tends to run in families.

Etiology

- Narcolepsy occurs because of a malfunction of the REM-inhibiting system.

Diagnosis

- NPSG will reveal REM periods that occur at sleep onset.
- MSLT will show excessive daytime sleepiness and increased REM sleep.

Course and Prognosis

- Narcolepsy is a chronic disease that requires lifelong treatment.

Treatment

- It is treated with CNS stimulants such as pemoline (Cylert) and methylphenidate (Ritalin).
- Afternoon naps may relieve daytime sleepiness.

Obstructive Sleep Apnea (continued)

OBSTRUCTIVE SLEEP APNEA

Epidemiology
- Sleep apnea may occur in up to one quarter of men and 10 percent of women.
- Prevalence statistics vary according to the study and sample population.
- It is more likely to occur in obese males.

Etiology
- Sleep apnea is a structural problem that involves an occlusion of the oropharynx.
- The obstruction is exacerbated when pharyngeal muscles relax during deep sleep.
- Central sleep apnea (not obstructive) occurs due to impaired respiratory drive during sleep.

Diagnosis
- NPSG will document the number and frequency of apneic events.
- An event is defined as 10 seconds or greater of breathing cessation and 30 events per night are required for diagnosis.
- MSLT may demonstrate daytime sleepiness associated with nighttime microawakenings.

Course and Prognosis
- Obstructive sleep apnea is a chronic disorder that requires lifelong treatment or surgery.

Treatment
- The treatment of choice for obstructive sleep apnea is continuous positive airway pressure (CPAP).
- Other treatments for obstructive sleep apnea are surgery (uvulopalatoplasty) and weight loss.
- Patients should not sleep in the supine position because it exacerbates the potential obstruction.

CIRCADIAN RHYTHM DISORDER

Epidemiology
- Jet-lag occurs in travelers, pilots, and airline crew.
- Shift-work disorder is frequent in physicians and people with constantly changing work schedules.
- Delayed sleep phase type is common in college students.

Etiology
- Causative factors vary according to the type of disturbance (e.g., travel, shift-work)

Diagnosis
- NPSG and MSLT may be helpful, but diagnosis can be based on the history alone.

Course and Prognosis
- Circadian rhythm disorders usually remit spontaneously when the causative factor is resolved.

Treatment
- Melatonin is used effectively for jet lag.
- Bright light therapy can treat delayed sleep phase disturbances.
- Proper sleep hygiene methods are used to promote alignment between external and circadian clocks.

SLEEP TERROR DISORDER

Epidemiology
- Sleep terrors are more likely to occur in children, boys in particular.

Etiology
- A neurological component such as temporal lobe pathology may play a role.
- Environmental factors such as anxiety also contribute.

Diagnosis
- Nighttime polysomnography.

Course and Prognosis
- Sleep terrors are usually transient and resolve spontaneously.
- They may be associated with temporal lobe epilepsy and enuresis.
- A sleep terror episode sometimes develops into a sleepwalking episode.

Treatment
- Night terrors are generally self-limited, but severe cases may require benzodiazepines.

NIGHTMARE DISORDER

Epidemiology
- Nightmares usually occur in young children and the incidence decreases with age.

Etiology
- Environmental stressors and anxiety are usually the cause of nightmares.

Diagnosis
- NPSG may be required to distinguish between sleep terrors and nightmares (non-REM vs. REM).

Course and Prognosis
- Nightmares are usually transient and resolve spontaneously.

Treatment
- Tricyclic antidepressants and benzodiazepines suppress REM sleep and may be effective in treating nightmares.

SLEEPWALKING DISORDER

Epidemiology
- Sleepwalking usually begins by age 8 and peak prevalence is at approximately 12 years old.

Etiology
- Sleepwalking tends to run in families.
- Neurological abnormalities may play a role.
- It may be associated with sleep terrors.

Diagnosis
- A description by parents or family members is sufficient for diagnosis.

Course and Prognosis
- Sleepwalking is usually transient and resolves spontaneously.

Treatment
- It is treated by waking the person from sleepwalking and averting the possibility of harm.

DIFFERENTIAL DIAGNOSIS

Medical
Sleep disorder due to a general medical condition: Neoplasm
Cardiovascular disease
Infection
Epilepsy
Cluster headache
Asthma
Gastroesophageal reflux

Psychiatric
Substance-induced sleep disorder (caffeine, alcohol, amphetamines, cocaine, opioids, and benzodiazepines)

Substance-Related Disorders: The Basics

IDENTIFICATION

There are 11 substance-related disorders but only the first 5 listed will be discussed:

1) Alcohol-related disorders
2) Cocaine-related disorders
3) Amphetamine-related disorders
4) Opioid-related disorders
5) Sedative/hypnotic/anxiolytic-related disorders
6) Caffeine-related disorders
7) Nicotine-related disorders
8) Cannabis-related disorders
9) Inhalant-related disorders
10) Hallucinogen-related disorders
11) Phencyclidine-related disorders

CHARACTERISTICS

Substance Abuse is characterized by at least **1** of the following:
1) Substance use causes a failure to fulfill major obligations at work, school, or home
2) Repeated use in situations where it is physically hazardous (e.g., driving)
3) Recurrent substance-related legal problems
4) Substance use continues despite psychological, medical, and interpersonal problems that result

Substance Dependence supersedes the diagnosis of abuse and is characterized by at least **3** of the following:
1) Tolerance
2) Withdrawal
3) Unintentionally excessive use
4) Efforts to control use persistently fail
5) Excessive time is spent trying to obtain the substance
6) Social, occupational, or recreational activities are reduced as a result of substance use
7) Use continues despite the knowledge of harmful effects

Substance-Related Disorders: Essential Features

REVIEW

Substance-related disorders are a vast topic and only a few of the specific substances will be covered in this section. Alcohol is the substance most frequently associated with abuse and dependence. Substance abuse becomes substance dependence when tolerance and withdrawal develop. Tolerance is defined as the need for increased amounts of the substance to produce the same effect. Withdrawal is defined as the presence of physical *or* psychological symptoms after cessation (or reduction) of a substance. This section will review the essential features of intoxication and withdrawal associated with 5 of the substance-related disorders.

ESSENTIAL FEATURES

Alcohol Intoxication
- The recent ingestion of alcohol may cause significant changes in behavior and functioning.
- The intoxicated individual may become **aggressive** or hypersexual.
- Mood may become **depressed** or labile (alcohol is considered a depressant).
- Physical signs of alcohol intoxication include **slurred speech,** incoordination, **unsteady gait,** nystagmus, impaired memory or attention, stupor or coma.
- Judgement and social/occupational functioning are impaired.

Alcohol Withdrawal
- Within several hours of stopping alcohol use patients may begin to **sweat,** and become **tachycardic.**
- **"The shakes"** (tremulousness) are the classic withdrawal sign and occur within 6 to 8 hours of alcohol cessation.
- **Psychotic symptoms** such as hallucinations (alcoholic hallucinosis) may occur within 8 to 12 hours.
- The classic hallucination associated with alcohol withdrawal is formication (ants crawling on the skin).
- **Seizures** can occur in alcohol withdrawal within 12 to 24 hours.
- **Delirium tremens** (alcohol withdrawal delirium) may begin anytime within 72 hours of alcohol cessation.
- Delirium tremens (DT) is characterized by **delirium** (e.g., perceptual disturbances, disorientation, agitation), **tremors,** and **fever.**
- Up to one third of patients who experience seizures during alcohol withdrawal go on to develop DTs.
- DTs typically only occur in patients who have abused alcohol for many years.

Cocaine Intoxication
- The recent use of cocaine is associated with specific affective and behavioral changes.
- Cocaine exerts its effects by increasing the concentration of dopamine available to dopamine receptors.
- Patients will appear manic with **elated mood,** a **heightened sense of self-esteem,** and **talkativeness.**
- Impaired judgement and impaired social/occupational functioning are common characteristics.
- Increased amounts of cocaine may produce tension, anxiety, and paranoia.
- Impulsive, aggressive, and hypersexual behavior is also frequently seen.
- Tactile hallucinations such as formication ("cocaine bugs") may occur.
- The physical signs of cocaine intoxication include **pupillary dilation, tachycardia,** and **hypertension.**
- Cocaine abusers may lose weight, have impaired concentration, and develop insomnia.
- Nasal congestion is a frequent finding due to rebound from the vasoconstrictive effects of the cocaine.
- The effects of cocaine resolve within 30 to 60 minutes.

Essential Features (continued)

Cocaine Withdrawal

- A post-intoxication depression is associated with cocaine withdrawal.
- Patients are **dysphoric, anhedonic, anxious,** and **irritable.**
- They may experience fatigue and hypersomnia with vivid, unpleasant dreams.
- Insomnia can also be seen.
- Psychomotor agitation *or* retardation can occur.
- Withdrawal symptoms are present for a day to a week, depending on the extent of use.

Amphetamine Intoxication

- The classic amphetamines are dextroamphetamine (Dexedrine), methamphetamine (Desoxyn), and methylphenidate (Ritalin).
- The street names of amphetamines are ice, crystal meth, and speed.
- Amphetamines act by increasing the release of catecholamines (particularly dopamine).
- The *designer* amphetamines have hallucinogenic properties because of dual action on serotonergic systems.
- The most common *designer* amphetamine is ecstasy [3,4-methylenedioxyamphetamine (MDMA)].
- Methcathinone (Crank) is a synthetic amphetamine that is made from over-the-counter preparations of ephedrine or pseudoephedrine.
- Amphetamine intoxication is very similar to cocaine intoxication because both substances increase the concentration of dopamine.
- Symptoms of mania such as **elated mood** and **pressured speech** are common features.
- **Tachycardia, pupillary dilation,** and **hypertension** are the typical physical signs.
- **Perceptual disturbances** are more likely to occur with amphetamines than with cocaine.
- The effects of amphetamines are mostly resolved within 24 hours.

Amphetamine Withdrawal

- The post-amphetamine crash includes symptoms of **dysphoria, anxiety,** and **fatigue.**
- Patients may be sweating with tremors, insomnia, or nightmares if they do sleep.
- Muscle and stomach cramps and hunger are also possible features.
- Withdrawal symptoms may last a week but usually peak within 2 to 4 days.

Opioid Intoxication

- Heroin is the most frequently abused opioid.
- Opioid intoxication is characterized by an initial **euphoria** followed by apathy.
- Patients may appear **slow** or **drowsy.**
- Memory and attention may be impaired.
- Judgement and social/occupational functioning are impaired.
- Physical signs are **miosis, slurred speech, respiratory depression,** and **hypothermia.**

Opioid Withdrawal

- There are 9 symptoms of opioid withdrawal: (1) **dysphoria,** (2) **nausea** or **vomiting,** (3) **muscle aches,** (4) **lacrimation** or **rhinorrhea,** (5) **pupillary dilation,** (6) **diarrhea,** (7) yawning, (8) fever, and (9) insomnia.
- Opioid withdrawal symptoms may occur within several hours of cessation and last days to weeks depending on the specific opioid abused.
- Withdrawal from heroin begins within 6 to 8 hours and lasts approximately 1 week.
- Withdrawal symptoms may be induced by administration of an opioid antagonist after opioid use.
- Asingle opioid injection immediately eliminates all withdrawal symptoms.

Essential Features (continued)

Sedative/Hypnotic/Anxiolytic Intoxication

- *Sedative* and *anxiolytic* are synonymous terms for drugs that **reduce anxiety.**
- Some of the sedative/anxiolytic drugs are also termed *hypnotic* because they **induce sleep.**
- **Benzodiazepines** and **barbiturates** are the main classes of drugs in the sedative/hypnotic/anxiolytic category.
- Benzodiazepines and barbiturates act on gamma-aminobutyric acid (GABA) receptors to increase their affinity to GABA.
- Benzodiazepines are schedule-IV controlled substances and *may* require a triplicate prescription depending on the state.
- Secobarbital (downers) is the most commonly known barbiturate.
- Methaqualone (quaaludes) is a barbiturate-like substance that is frequently abused.
- Flunitrazepam (roofies) is the benzodiazepine associated with date rape and is illegal in the U.S.
- Benzodiazepine and barbiturate intoxication is very similar to alcohol intoxication.
- Symptoms include **behavioral disinhibition** with slurred speech, incoordination, nystagmus, impaired concentration and memory, and possibly stupor or coma.
- Benzodiazepines may elicit aggressive behavior particularly if combined with alcohol.
- Benzodiazepines are not as frequently associated with euphoria as barbiturates.
- Barbiturates cause the same intoxication syndrome as alcohol and benzodiazepines, but are more likely to induce feelings of euphoria.
- **Respiratory depression** is a potentially fatal effect of sedative/hypnotic/anxiolytic use.

Sedative/Hypnotic/Anxiolytic Withdrawal

- Withdrawal from benzodiazepines and especially barbiturates may be life-threatening and require hospitalization.
- Barbiturates are associated with a more dangerous withdrawal syndrome than benzodiazepines because of the risk of sudden death.
- There are 8 withdrawal symptoms of sedative/hypnotic/anxiolytic abuse: (1)**autonomic hyperactivity** (2) **hand tremors,** (3) **insomnia,** (4) **nausea** or **vomiting,** (5) **hallucinations,** (6) **psychomotor agitation,** (7) **anxiety,** and (8) **seizures.**
- Autonomic hyperactivity includes **sweating** and **tachycardia** (>100 bpm).
- Hallucinations may be visual, tactile, or auditory, and are transient.
- Seizures are typically the grand mal type.
- Withdrawal symptoms occur 2 or 3 days after cessation depending on the specific drug.
- Diazepam (Valium) has a very long half-life and withdrawal symptoms may not appear for 5 to 6 days.
- Withdrawal symptoms should be avoided by tapering the dosage slowly.

Substance-Related Disorders: Depth and Detail

REVIEW

Substance abuse and dependence frequently co-exist with psychiatric disorders. In some cases psychiatric illness may be the direct result of a substance-related disorder. Patients that suffer from a substance-related disorder *and* a psychiatric illness independent of the substance abuse are termed "dual-diagnosis." This section will review the details of 5 important substance-related disorders.

ALCOHOL

Epidemiology
- Alcohol is the most commonly abused substance.
- Approximately 10 percent of women and 20 percent of men meet the criteria for alcohol *abuse.*
- Approximately 5 percent of women and 10 percent meet the criteria for alcohol *dependence.*

Etiology
- A combination of psychosocial and genetic factors contribute to the development of alcohol abuse.
- People are more likely to abuse alcohol in settings where drinking is socially acceptable (e.g., college)
- First-degree relatives of alcohol abusers show increased rates of alcohol-related disorders.
- Twin studies have revealed a partial genetic basis for alcohol-related disorders, particularly in men.

Diagnosis
- The **C.A.G.E questionnaire** is frequently used to determine the extent of alcohol use.
- Ask the patient if they have ever: (1) tried to **Cut** down alcohol use, (2) felt **Annoyed** by people criticizing their drinking, (3) felt **Guilty** about drinking, or (4) had a morning **Eye-opener.**
- If patients answer yes to 2 of the C.A.G.E. questions it raises the suspicion of alcohol dependence.
- If they answer yes to all 4 C.A.G.E. questions it's considered pathognomonic for dependence.
- Physical signs of alcohol abuse include palmar erythema, acne rosacea, and painless hepatomegaly (fatty liver).
- Patients who abuse alcohol may have an elevated mean corpuscular erythrocyte volume.
- Signs of more advanced disease are secondary to liver cirrhosis and include jaundice, ascites, gynecomastia, testicular atrophy, and Duputyren's contracture.
- Intoxication is confirmed by serum toxicology screen and blood alcohol levels.

Complications
- Blackouts (anterograde amnesia), car accidents, and arrests for driving under the influence frequently complicate the course of alcohol abuse.
- Medical complications of alcohol abuse/dependence include liver disease, cardiomyopathy, electrolyte imbalance, respiratory depression, and fetal alcohol syndrome during pregnancy.
- In severe cases alcohol can induce dementia, amnesia, psychotic disorders, mood disorders, and anxiety disorders.
- Wernicke-Korsakoff syndrome is caused by thiamine deficiency and is commonly associated with alcohol dependence.
- **Wernicke's** encephalopathy consists of acute, *reversible* symptoms of **nystagmus, ataxia,** and **mental confusion.**

Alcohol (continued)

- **Korsakoff's** psychosis is *irreversible* in 75 percent of patients and consists of **anterograde amnesia** and **confabulation.**

Treatment

- Suspected alcohol-dependent patients should be treated *prophylactically* with chlordiazepoxide (Librium) or lorazepam (Ativan) to avoid withdrawal symptoms.
- Oral supplementation of thiamine and folate is given to prevent Wernicke-Korsakoff syndrome.
- "The shakes" (tremulousness) are treated with chlordiazepoxide.
- Psychotic symptoms such as alcoholic hallucinosis are treated with lorazepam or antipsychotics.
- Withdrawal seizures are treated with diazepam (Valium).
- Delirium tremens is treated with lorazepam.
- Alcohol rehabilitation is achieved through support groups that encourage abstinence.
- Alcoholics Anonymous (AA) is a 12-step outpatient program that is effective in maintaining sobriety.
- Inpatient and residential rehabilitation programs also exist.
- Group therapy is the psychotherapeutic method of choice.
- Pharmacotherapy treatments include disulfiram (Antabuse) and naltrexone (ReVia), and SSRI studies are currently underway.
- Treatment of associated psychiatric symptoms should be considered only after several weeks of sobriety to ensure that symptoms are not directly caused by alcohol use.

COCAINE

Epidemiology

- Cocaine users represent less than 1 percent of the population.
- The recent decrease in the use of powder cocaine has been offset by an increase in crack cocaine use.

Mechanism of Action

- Cocaine acts by competitive inhibition of dopamine reuptake.
- The concentration of dopamine available to dopamine receptors is increased.
- The effects of cocaine are felt immediately and last for 30 to 60 minutes.
- Cocaine powder may be inhaled through the nose or injected intravenously.
- Crack cocaine is the pure cocaine alkaloid form (freebase) that is smoked.
- Crack cocaine is more potent, more addictive, and less expensive than powder cocaine.
- Cocaine metabolites remain in the blood and urine for approximately 10 days.

Complications

- The adverse effects of cocaine use include nasal congestion, cerebrovascular effects, seizures, cardiac effects, and sudden death.
- **Nasal congestion** is a result of rebound vasodilation from the vasoconstriction, and swelling, bleeding, and ulceration may also occur.
- In extreme cases with chronic abuse, the nasal septum may become perforated.
- **Cerebrovascular** effects include cerebral infarctions and hemorrhages from vasoconstriction.
- Cocaine is the substance of abuse most likely to cause **seizures.**
- **Cardiac** effects include myocardial infarction and cardiac arrhythmias.
- Cocaine abuse may lead to psychiatric complications such as delirium, psychosis, mood disorders, and anxiety disorders.

Cocaine (continued)

Treatment

- Initial treatment is focused on diminishing the patient's craving for the substance.
- Cognitive-behavioral therapy may be effective.
- Individual therapy will focus on the patient's initial motives in beginning the substance abuse.
- Group therapy and support groups like Narcotics Anonymous may facilitate long-term abstinence.
- Pharmacologic treatments include dopamine agonists and tricyclic antidepressants to reduce craving.
- Methylphenidate (Ritalin) has been used effectively to help patients cope with withdrawal symptoms.

AMPHETAMINES

Epidemiology

- Amphetamines are most commonly abused by 18 to 25 year olds.
- Approximately one percent of the population use amphetamines.
- Amphetamines are *abused* to produce feelings of **euphoria,** to increase **performance** in students, to increase **endurance** in athletes, and to **suppress appetite.**
- They are also are used medically to increase concentration in ADHD.

Mechanism of Action

- Amphetamines act by increasing the release of catecholamines from presynaptic nerve terminals.
- The dopaminergic neurons are particularly affected and account for the addictive component.
- Designer amphetamines such as MDMA (ecstasy) increase the release of both catecholamines and serotonin.
- The serotonergic effects account for the hallucinogenic properties of designer amphetamines.
- Amphetamines are present in the urine for 1 to 2 days.

Complications

- Amphetamine abuse is associated with amphetamine-induced psychotic disorder, mood disorder, anxiety disorder, sexual dysfunction, and sleep disorder.

Treatment

- Treatment options are psychotherapeutic and pharmacologic.
- Cognitive-behavioral therapy, group therapy, and support groups such as Narcotics Anonymous may be effective.
- Benzodiazepines are used to treat agitation and hyperactivity associated with amphetamine withdrawal.

OPIOIDS

Epidemiology

- Heroin is the opioid that is most frequently associated with abuse and dependence.
- Less than 0.2% of the population is dependent on heroin.
- Tolerance and dependence develop very quickly in opioid (particularly heroin) use.

Mechanism of Action

- Opioids act on specific opioid receptors in the brain.
- These receptors regulate analgesia, dependence, respiratory depression, constipation, and sedation.
- Opioids also act on dopaminergic and noradrenergic neurotransmitter systems.
- Heroin is very lipid soluble and easily passes the blood brain barrier so its effects are felt immediately.
- Opioids are present in the urine and blood for 12 to 36 hours.

Opioids (continued)

Complications
- Intravenous use of opioids is associated with increased rates of transmission of HIV and hepatitis.
- Opioids cause respiratory depression, and an overdose can result in respiratory arrest.
- Heroin abuse during pregnancy is associated with miscarriage, fetal death, and neonatal withdrawal.
- Opioid abuse and dependence may also induce delirium, psychotic disorder, mood disorder, sleep disorder, and sexual dysfunction.

Treatment
- Methadone maintenance is often used to manage patients with heroin dependence.
- Methadone is an opioid that is taken orally to suppress heroin withdrawal symptoms without producing euphoria.
- Methadone must be administered daily but it does not impair social and occupational functioning.
- It is easier to wean patients from methadone than heroin.
- Clonidine (Catapres) is used to reduce withdrawal symptoms from methadone.
- Opioid overdose is treated with the opioid antagonists naloxone (Narcan) and naltrexone (ReVia).

SEDATIVE/HYPNOTIC/ANXIOLYTICS

Epidemiology
- Sedative/hypnotic/anxiolytic drugs account for approximately 25 percent of substance-related emergency room visits.
- Benzodiazepines in particular are frequently (but unsuccessfully) used in suicide attempts.

Mechanism of Action
- Barbiturates and benzodiazepines bind the type A gamma-aminobutyric acid (GABA) receptor complex.
- They increase the receptor's affinity for GABA, an *inhibitory* neurotransmitter.

Complications
- Benzodiazepines have a large margin of safety and huge doses are required for overdose.
- The combination of benzodiazepines and alcohol can be lethal.
- Less severe complications of benzodiazepine overdose are lethargy, ataxia, and confusion.
- Barbiturates cause **respiratory depression** more easily than benzodiazepines.
- An overdose of barbiturates leads to respiratory arrest, coma, and death.
- Tolerance to barbiturates develops quickly, and over time toxic doses may be required to produce the desired effect.
- Patients do *not* develop tolerance to the side effects of respiratory depression and arrest.
- Accidental overdoses of barbiturates may occur, particularly in children.

Treatment
- Benzodiazepine taper must be gradual, and carbamazepine (Tegretol) may be used to prevent seizures.
- Benzodiazepine overdose is treated with flumazenil (Romazicon), a benzodiazepine antagonist.
- Barbiturate withdrawal may cause sudden death, and a slow taper is also required.
- Phenobarbital is substituted for the abused barbiturate during the tapering period.
- Barbiturate overdose is treated with gastric lavage and charcoal to delay absorption.
- Outpatient support is necessary to help patients remain free of benzodiazepine and barbiturate use.

Suicide

SUICIDE is the successful and intentional attempt to end one's life.

Clinical Features
- Suicide is usually the result of feelings of depression and hopelessness that become unbearable.
- The patient will feel that the only escape from their suffering is death.
- The best indicator of suicidal risk is past suicidal behavior.
- Feelings of **hopelessness** is another reliable predictor for increased risk of suicide.
- Suicide is more likely to occur in patients who are just recovering from suicidal depression and treatment of depression may supply the energy to act that the patient previously lacked.
- Risk factors include increased age (>45), alcohol dependence, prior violent or suicidal behavior, depression, medical or psychiatric illness, unemployment, recent divorce or loss of a loved one, and family history of suicide.

Epidemiology
- Women are more likely to attempt suicide and men are more likely to succeed.
- Women often use drug overdoses and men use more violent means (e.g., shooting, hanging, jumping).
- Suicide is the ninth overall cause of death in the United States.
- Suicide rates among adolescents have increased significantly in recent decades.
- Suicide is most frequently associated with major depression.
- Approximately 15 percent of patients with major depression eventually commit suicide.
- Approximately one-third of patients with schizophrenia will attempt suicide and 10 percent will succeed.

Etiology
- Suicide is associated with psychological and biological factors.
- Freud believed that suicide was homicidal or aggressive tendencies turned inward.
- More recent theories include beliefs of self-punishment, revenge, escape, or reunion with the dead.
- Family members of suicide victims are at a higher risk.
- Suicide by violent methods is associated with *decreased* serotonin metabolism as measured by de*creased* serotonin metabolite (5HIAA) in the cerebrospinal fluid (CSF).
- *Decreased* 5HIAA in the CSF is associated with impulsive and aggressive behavior in general.

Diagnosis
- Suicidal ideation should always be evaluated in a mental status exam.
- Many patients will reveal thoughts about suicide prior to attempts.
- The presence of a specific "plan" greatly increases the risk of suicide.
- Risk factors for suicide need to be assessed in conjunction with any psychiatric complaints.
- The physician should always ask about family history of suicide and prior attempts.

Treatment (continued)

Treatment

- Inpatient hospitalization is usually required for suicide attempts.
- Hospitalization is also required for suicidal thoughts if there is a lack of social support, previous suicide attempts, or a specific plan.
- Suicidal patients can only be treated on an outpatient basis if they agree to contact their psychiatrist if they doubt their ability to control suicidal impulses.
- Psychiatrists need to be available to the suicidal outpatient at all times.
- Family members should be notified.
- Underlying medical or psychiatric conditions must be appropriately addressed.

Child Abuse

CHILD ABUSE is defined as mistreatment by physical abuse, sexual abuse, emotional abuse, or child neglect.

Clinical Features
- Children who have been **physically abused** show multiple bruises that cannot be adequately explained.
- Physically abused children may appear withdrawn, frightened, or overly aggressive.
- Their mood may be depressed or labile, and anxiety or paranoid ideation may be observed.
- Cigarette burns, spiral fractures, and retinal hemorrhages from shaking should raise suspicion of abuse.
- Children who are **sexually abused** may seem precocious, and have explicit knowledge of sexual acts.
- They may interact with peers using inappropriate sexual behavior.
- Victims of sexual abuse may feel shame, guilt, and excessive fear of adults.
- Physical signs of sexual abuse include genital pain, bleeding and itching, recurrent urinary tract infections, and vaginal discharge or the presence of a sexually transmitted disease.
- **Neglect of a child** involves failure to thrive, poor hygiene, hunger, and chronic infections.
- Neglected children may be socially withdrawn or inappropriately affectionate with strangers.
- Evidence of physical abuse is usually not present in cases of child neglect.

Epidemiology
- Every year in the U.S. 2,000 to 4,000 deaths occur because of child abuse or neglect.
- Approximately 1 out of 4 girls and 1out of 8 boys will be sexually abused by the time they are 18.
- Abused or neglected children are more likely to have been premature or low birth weight neonates.
- Mentally retarded or physically disabled children are at a higher risk of being abused.
- Perpetrators of sexual abuse are usually known to the victim (e.g., parent, uncle, sibling, friend).
- The risk of developing depressive disorders, anxiety disorders, posttraumatic stress disorder, aggressive behavior, and suicidal behavior are all increased in children who were physically abused.
- Children who were sexually abused are more likely to develop dissociative disorders, borderline personality disorder, or substance-related disorders.

Etiology
- The vast majority of children are abused by parents who were abused themselves.
- Families of abused children are more frequently living in a stressful environment (e.g., marital conflict, single-parent household, poverty).
- Parents who are substance abusers are at increased risk of committing child abuse or neglect.
- Hyperactive children may be abused as a form of discipline.

Diagnosis
- Physical abuse must be suspected if injuries have inconsistent or poorly explained causes.
- A history of multiple injuries or old scars should increase suspicion.
- Bruises that form symmetrical patterns (cigarette burns) or affect both sides of the face or body indicate physical abuse.
- Spiral fractures or retinal hemorrhage in an infant are classic signs of probable physical abuse.
- Genital pain, itching, bleeding, or discharge are signs of sexual abuse.
- Pediatricians should suspect sexual abuse in cases of sexually transmitted disease and recurrent urinary tract infections in young children.

Treatment

- Physicians must report all cases of physical abuse, sexual abuse, or child neglect to the appropriate social service department as soon as the diagnosis is made.
- Psychologists, school personnel, hospital staff, and police are also *mandated* to report child abuse.
- The child's immediate safety is the first goal of treatment.
- A complete psychiatric and physical exam should be performed.
- Intervention for the child and family must be arranged with social services.

Forensic Psychiatry

REVIEW

Forensic psychiatry is concerned with mental disorders as they relate to the legal system. Examples of legal issues include competency hearings, criminal responsibility, and malpractice litigation. This section will review the terms and definitions that it is necessary to be familiar with in the field of forensic psychiatry.

PRIVILEGE

- Privilege is the right to maintain confidentiality within the confines of a protected relationship.
- Communication between physicians and patients is considered privileged information.
- The law *may* protect the physician against forced disclosure under the circumstances of a subpoena.
- The right of privilege belongs only to the patient, and *not* to the physician.
- Physicians are *not* legally entitled to the same privilege that exists between attorneys and clients, husbands and wives, or rabbis and members of the congregation.
- Medical privilege does *not* exist in military courts, criminal responsibility hearings, hospitalization hearings, malpractice suits, or child-custody and child-protection proceedings.

CONFIDENTIALITY

- Confidentiality refers to the obligation of physicians to hold all patient information secret.
- Information may only be shared with other staff members, clinical supervisors, or medical consultants.
- The physician must receive permission from the patient to share information with family members, previous physicians, and legal personnel unless it is deemed an emergency situation.
- Confidentiality may be breached in cases of potential or actual child abuse.
- **Tarasoff I** (*duty to warn*) is a court ruling that allows a therapist to breach confidentiality and notify the police if:
  1) A patient will probably commit murder.
  2) A patient will probably commit suicide.
  3) A patient with life-threatening responsibilities (e.g., pilots) shows marked impairment of judgement.
- **Tarasoff II** (*duty to protect*) broadened Tarasoff I to rule that confidentiality may also be breached in cases where a patient makes an *explicit* threat of violence against a specific person.

INFORMED CONSENT

- A patient has the right to appropriate information regarding all aspects of a proposed treatment.
- The patient must be able to understand the risks and benefits of the proposed treatment.
- The patient must give consent voluntarily.
- In the case of a minor, the parent or guardian must give consent unless it is an emergency.
- Minors do *not* need parental consent for prenatal care, abortion, alcohol and drug abuse, and sexually transmitted disease.

MALPRACTICE

- Malpractice occurs when a physician's failure to perform his duty directly causes damage.
- Malpractice is defined legally by the Four Ds: **Dereliction, Duty, Direct** and **Damage.**
- **Dereliction** is the failure to perform according to the "average standard of care" in treating the patient.
- **Duty** refers to the obligation of the physician to provide proper care of the patient.
- **Direct** means that the physician's negligence (dereliction) *directly* caused the alleged damage.
- **Damage** must be shown to have occurred.
- Suicide and suicide attempts are the number one reasons for malpractice suits against psychiatrists.
- Psychiatry ranks eighth among medical specialties in frequency of malpractice suits.

HOSPITALIZATION

- "Hospitalization" is the term that has replaced "commitment" for an involuntary hospital admission.
- Involuntary admission occurs when there is a risk of suicide or homicide.
- There must be evidence that the patient is either a **danger to self or to others.**
- In some states, hospitalization is also warranted if the patient is **unable to care for him or herself.**
- Involuntary patients have the right to refuse treatment unless they are declared incompetent by a court.
- The patient may appeal the involuntary status and bring the case before a judge.
- Kendra's law (1999) mandates assisted outpatient treatment (AOT) for people with mental illness who would not comply with treatment without strict supervision.
- Kendra's law requires inpatient "hospitalization" for patients who do not comply with AOT.
- Petitioning a court for AOT may be done by the patient's roommate, parent, spouse, adult child, psychiatrist, hospital director, community program director, or parole/probation officer.

COMPETENCE TO STAND TRIAL

- Someone who is mentally incompetent is prohibited from standing trial in the United States.
- Competence is defined as a "rational" and "factual" understanding of the proceedings *and* charges.
- There are clinical guides that identify areas of functioning and are used to determine competence.
- Mental illness alone is not sufficient to deem someone incompetent.
- Competence in general is judged based on the patient's understanding of the specific issues involved.
- Psychiatrists can only offer clinical opinions about competency, it is the judge who decides legally.

CRIMINAL RESPONSIBILITY

- An objectionable act is only defined as a crime if there are two components: voluntary conduct (*actus reus*) and evil intent (*mens rea*).
- The theory is that someone who is mentally ill does not understand the nature of the objectionable act and therefore could not have had evil intent.
- Voluntary conduct *without* evil intent does not qualify as a crime and *therefore* the mentally ill should not be prosecuted as criminals.

- The **M'Naughten Rule** (1843) states that a person is not guilty by reason of insanity if they suffered from a mental illness that precluded them from understanding the nature and consequences of the act, or prevented them from understanding that the act was wrong.
- **Irresistible Impulse** (1922) is referred to as the policeman-at-the-elbow law where a person is not responsible for an act that was committed under an impulse that was irresistible due to mental disease.
- The **Model Penal Code** (1962) is recommended today by the American Law Institute and states that people are not responsible for criminal conduct if they lack the capacity [due to mental disease] to appreciate the "wrongfulness" of their conduct or are unable to change their conduct according to the requirements of the law.

Antipsychotics: The Basics

IDENTIFICATION

There are two classes of antipsychotic medication: **dopamine receptor antagonists** and **serotonin-dopamine antagonists.** Dopamine receptor antagonists were previously called "typical" and serotonin-dopamine antagonists were called "atypical." Dopamine receptor antagonists are further divided into 3 categories of low, mid, and high-potency.

Low-potency dopamine receptor antagonists

*Chlorpromazine (Thorazine)

*Thioridazine (Mellaril)

Mesoridazine (Serentil)

Mid-potency dopamine receptor antagonists

*Perphenazine (Trilafon)

Loxapine (Loxitane)

Molindone (Moban)

High-potency dopamine receptor antagonists

*Haloperidol (Haldol)

*Fluphenazine (Prolixin)

*Pimozide (Orap)

Trifluoperazine (Stelazine)

Serotonin-dopamine antagonists

*Clozapine (Clozaril)

*Quetiapine (Seroquel)

*Risperidone (Risperidal)

*Olanzapine (Zyprexa)

Sertindole (Serlect)

Ziprasidone (Geodon)

---

*It is important to be most familiar with the antipsychotics marked by an asterisk.

CHARACTERISTICS

Dopamine receptor antagonists decrease dopaminergic activity by blocking mainly dopamine 2 (D2) receptors. They may be equally effective as serotonin-dopamine antagonists in treating the **positive** symptoms of psychosis (e.g., hallucinations). However, dopamine receptor antagonists are associated with an *increased* risk of extrapyramidal-related side effects as compared to the serotonin-dopamine antagonists.

Serotonin-dopamine antagonists decrease dopaminergic activity *and* serotonergic activity by antagonism at D2 and serotonin 2A receptors. They may be more effective than dopamine receptor antagonists for treatment-resistant psychosis and the negative symptoms of psychosis (e.g., affective flattening). Serotonin-dopamine antagonists are *less* likely to be associated with extrapyramidal side effects.

REVIEW

The Dopamine Hypothesis is the model for antipsychotic treatment and it posits that excessive dopaminergic activity is the underlying cause for psychotic states. There are two main classifications of antipsychotic medication: dopamine receptor antagonists act mainly on dopamine 2 (D2) receptors, and serotonin-dopamine antagonists have combined serotonergic effects by blockade of serotonin 2A (5HT2A) and D2 receptors. Antipsychotic medications differ in their potency, their selectivity for specific dopamine receptor sites, and their additional effects on cholinergic, adrenergic, and histaminergic systems. This section will review the mechanism of action, indications, and side effects of the antipsychotics.

DOPAMINE RECEPTOR ANTAGONISTS

Mechanism of Action

- Dopamine receptor antagonists are thought to exert their effect by dopaminergic blockade of the pathways from the midbrain to the prefrontal cortex (mesocortical) and limbic system (mesolimbic).
- High-potency antipsychotics have the highest affinity for D2 receptors.
- Low-potency antipsychotics bind D2 receptors with a lower affinity and are more likely to affect cholinergic, adrenergic, and histaminergic systems.

Indications

- All **psychotic disorders** may be treated with dopamine receptor antagonists.
- **Major depression with psychotic features**
- **Acute mania**
- **Tourette's disorder** can be treated with haloperidol (Haldol) or pimozide (Orap).
- **Huntington's chorea** may be effectively treated with haloperidol.
- Psychotic symptoms associated with **dementia** or **substance abuse** may be treated with high-potency antipsychotics.

Side Effects

- High-potency dopamine receptor antagonists cause more extrapyramidal side effects (EPS) because of increased D2 blockade and *reduced* dopaminergic activity.
- Low-potency medications are more likely to have anticholinergic, antiadrenergic, and antihistaminergic side effects.
- Cholinergic antagonism is protective against EPS because it *increases* dopamine release.
- **Extrapyramidal** side effects are parkinsonism, dystonia, tardive dyskinesia, akathisia, and neuroleptic malignant syndrome (see "Extrapyramidal Symptoms" chapter for a full discussion).
- **Anticholinergic** side effects are dry mouth, urinary retention, constipation, and blurred vision.
- **Antiadrenergic** side effects are orthostatic hypotension, tachycardia, and sexual dysfunction.
- **Antihistaminergic** side effects are weight gain, sedation, and fatigue.
- Thioridazine (low-potency) can cause **pigmentary retinopathy** or **retrograde ejaculation.**
- Dopamine receptor antagonism may cause **increased serum prolactin** levels and in some cases lead to galactorrhea, amenorrhea, or impotence in men.

Serotonin-Dopamine Antagonists (continued)

SEROTONIN-DOPAMINE ANTAGONISTS

Mechanism of Action

- Serotonin-dopamine antagonists reduce dopaminergic activity *and* serotonergic activity by D2 and 5HT-2A receptor blockade.
- Dopamine blockade may also occur at D1 and D4 receptors (e.g., clozapine and olanzapine).
- Serotonin-dopamine antagonists may act more selectively on the mesolimbic and mesocortical dopaminergic system, the proposed site of antipsychotic action.
- A lower affinity for the nigrostriatal dopamine pathway results in far fewer extrapyramidal side effects.
- Adrenergic, cholinergic, and histaminergic systems can also be affected.

Indications

- All **psychotic disorders**
- **Acute mania**
- **Major depression with psychotic features**
- Psychotic symptoms associated with **dementia,** or **substance abuse.**
- **Negative symptoms** that do not respond to dopamine receptor antagonists may be effectively treated with serotonin-dopamine antagonists.
- **Treatment-resistant** schizophrenia may respond to clozapine in approximately 30 percent of cases.

Side Effects

- Extrapyramidal side effects are infrequent with serotonin-dopamine antagonists.
- The major adverse effects of clozapine are **agranulocytosis** and an increased risk for **seizures.**
- Other side effects of clozapine are **sedation** (histamine blockade), **constipation** (cholinergic blockade), and **hypotension** and increased salivation (alpha blockade).
- The main side effects of quetiapine are **hypotension, sedation, weight gain,** and **dyspepsia.**
- Risperidone is associated with **sedation, increased prolactin levels,** and **prolonged QT.**
- Olanzapine has adverse effects of **sedation, constipation,** and **weight gain.**

Table: Distinguishing Characteristics of Dopamine Receptor Antagonists

Drug	Potency	EPS	Anticholinergic	Sedative	Hypotensive
Chlorpromazine	Low	Low	Medium	High	High
Thioridazine	Low	Low	High	High	High
Perphenazine	Medium	High	Low	Low	Low
Haloperidol	High	High	Low	Low	Low
Fluphenazine	High	High	Low	Medium	Low
Pimozide	High	High	Low	Low	Low

Table: Distinguishing Characteristics of Serotonin-Dopamine Antagonists

Drug	Potency	EPS	Anticholinergic	Sedative	Hypotensive
Clozapine	Low	None	High	High	High
Quetiapine	Low	None	Low	Medium	Medium
Olanzapine	High	Low	Medium	Medium	Medium
Risperidone	High	Low	Low	Low	Low

Adapted from Hyman SE, Arana GW, Rosenbaum JF: *Handbook of Psychiatric Drug Therapy,* Fourth Edition.

REVIEW

Dopamine receptor antagonists are very effective medications for treating positive symptoms of psychosis. They are not as well tolerated as the serotonin-dopamine antagonists, however, and they do not address the negative symptoms of psychosis. Serotonin-dopamine antagonists are more effective in treating negative symptoms and are much less frequently associated with extrapyramidal side effects. The cost of serotonin-dopamine antagonists may be prohibitive and their use is sometimes reserved for after typical dopamine-receptor antagonists fail or are not tolerated. This section reviews the pharmacokinetics, dosage and administration, and precautions of both classes of antipsychotics.

DOPAMINE RECEPTOR AND SEROTONIN-DOPAMINE ANTAGONISTS

Pharmacokinetics

- The half-lives of antipsychotics range from 10 to 20 hours.
- Haloperidol (Haldol) and fluphenazine (Prolixin) are available in long-acting parenteral (depot) forms.
- Peak plasma concentrations are reached 1 to 4 hours after oral administration (depending on the antipsychotic) and within 1 hour after intramuscular injection.
- Antipsychotics are metabolized by the liver.

Dosage and Administration

- Antipsychotic effects occur within 1 to 2 weeks of administration.
- Sedating effects occur within 1 hour of administration and last several hours.
- The equivalent of 8–12 mg/day of haloperidol (high-potency) is generally sufficient for an adult (400–600 mg/day of low-potency chlorpromazine).
- Elderly patients require lower doses of antipsychotics.
- *Acute* psychotic agitation is generally treated with haloperidol.
- *Non*-psychotic agitation is better treated with chlorpromazine because it is more sedating and has fewer extrapyramidal side effects than haloperidol (benzodiazepines are another option).
- Haloperidol decanoate and fluphenazine decanoate are long-acting depot preparations given IM every 2–4 weeks for patients who are non-compliant with oral administration.
- Clozapine requires weekly CBC monitoring for agranulocytosis.
- Maintenance antipsychotic treatment should continue for 1–2 years after the first psychotic episode.
- Treatment should continue for 5 years after a second psychotic episode, and lifelong after a third.

Dopamine Receptor and Serotonin-Dopamine Antagonists (continued)

Precautions

- Antipsychotics should not be used if there is a history of **allergic reaction** to such agents.
- Antipsychotics are contraindicated with **substance intoxication** (alcohol, opioid, barbiturate, and benzodiazepine) because of CNS depression.
- **Anticholinergic delirium** is a contraindication to antipsychotic administration.
- **Cardiac abnormalities** must be considered because antipsychotics may induce cardiac arrhythmias.
- Pimozide cannot be administered with **macrolide antibiotics** (erythromycin, clarithromycin, azithromycin, and dirithromycin) because of cardiac toxicity.
- Low-potency dopamine antagonists and clozapine reduce the seizure threshold and may be contraindicated in **seizure disorders.**
- Clozapine is contraindicated if white blood cells (WBCs) are less than 3,500 per mm^3.
- Clozapine cannot be used with other medications that cause agranulocytosis (e.g., carbamazepine).
- Anticholinergic side effects may exacerbate symptoms of **prostatic hypertrophy** (e.g., urinary retention).

Extrapyramidal Symptoms

REVIEW

The DSM-IV classifies extrapyramidal symptoms as Neuroleptic-Induced Movement Disorders. "Neuroleptic" is an old term that referred to typical antipsychotics. Typical antipsychotics are now called "dopamine receptor antagonists." There are 5 extrapyramidal symptoms associated with dopamine receptor antagonists: **parkinsonism, neuroleptic malignant syndrome, acute dystonia, acute akathisia,** and **tardive dyskinesia.** Extrapyramidal symptoms are reduced with low-potency dopamine receptor antagonists and are very rare with the newer serotonin-dopamine antagonists.

PARKINSONISM

Clinical Features
- Neuroleptic-induced parkinsonism is characterized by tremor, rigidity, and bradykinesia.
- The **tremor** occurs at rest (i.e., resting tremor) and oscillates at a rate of 3–6 cycles per second.
- **Rigidity** refers to increased muscle tone and is defined as increased resistance to passive movement.
- Parkinsonian rigidity is described as either lead-pipe or cogwheel type.
- Lead-pipe rigidity is increased tone throughout the range of motion.
- Cogwheel rigidity is increased tone with a superimposed jerkiness.
- **Bradykinesia** is characterized by (1) difficulty in initiating movement, (2) decreased arm-swing while walking, (3) shuffling gait, and (4) a mask-like facial expression.
- A mask-like facial expression may also occur as a negative symptom of schizophrenia (flat affect).

Epidemiology
- Neuroleptic-induced parkinsonism occurs most frequently in **elderly women.**
- It is most likely to occur **after several weeks** of therapy.

Etiology
- Dopamine 2 receptor blockade in the nigrostriatal dopamine pathway.

Treatment
- Reduce the dosage of the antispychotic.
- Give anticholinergic medications benztropine (Cogentin) or trihexyphenidyl (Artane).
- Consider switching to a serotonin-dopamine receptor antagonist.
- Prophylactic anticholinergic treatment may be considered before parkinsonism appears.

NEUROLEPTIC MALIGNANT SYNDROME (NMS)

Clinical Features

- NMS is characterized by (1) autonomic instability, (2) motor problems, and (3) behavioral disturbance.
- **Autonomic instability** includes hypertension, tachycardia, and hyperpyrexia.
- **Motor problems** are *rigidity, dystonia,* akinesia, and mutism.
- **Behavioral disturbance** includes agitation, incontinence, delirium, seizures, and coma.
- Laboratory tests may reveal **increased creatine kinase** from muscular rigidity, **abnormal liver function tests,** and **leukocytosis.**
- NMS may be fatal in 20 to 30 percent of patients who develop it.
- Serotonin syndrome (see "Antidepressants" chapter) may appear similar to NMS but does *not* include symptoms of *muscle rigidity* and *dystonia.*

Epidemiology

- The major risk factor for NMS is **high doses** of dopamine receptor antagonists.
- It is more common in **young men.**
- NMS may occur **at any point** during antipsychotic treatment.

Etiology

- NMS is considered an idiosyncratic reaction, and the pathophysiology is unclear.

Treatment

- The first step of treatment is withdrawal of the antipsychotic agent.
- Intravenous fluids should be started immediately.
- Intravenous dantrolene (calcium channel blocker) is given as a muscle relaxant.
- Bromocriptine (dopamine agonist) is used to counter the dopamine receptor blockade.
- Later switch to a serotonin-dopamine antagonist.

ACUTE DYSTONIA

Clinical Features

- Dystonia is a brief spasm or prolonged contraction of muscles, most often of the head and neck.
- Dystonic reactions result in abnormal and sometimes bizarre postures or movements.
- Examples include tongue protrusion, torticollis, oculogyric crisis, drooling from pharyngeal spasm, and limb/trunk muscle contraction.
- Laryngeal muscle spasms may produce airway compromise.

Epidemiology

- The major risk factor for acute dystonia is **high doses** of **high-potency** dopamine-receptor antagonists.
- It occurs most often in **young men** (<40 years old).
- Dystonic reactions usually appear within the **first few days** of antipsychotic treatment.

Etiology

- Dystonia is proposed to result from changes in dopaminergic activity within the basal ganglia as dopamine-receptor blockade wears off in between doses.

Acute Dystonia (continued)

Treatment

- Immediate treatment with intramuscular anticholinergic medication is necessary.
- Intravenous anticholinergics are used in severe cases.
- The most effective treatment for focal dystonia is botulinum toxin.
- Intubation may be required if larnyngospasm causes severe respiratory distress.
- Antipsychotic treatment may continue with standing adjuvant anticholinergic medication.
- Switching antipsychotic medication is not always necessary.

ACUTE AKATHISIA

Clinical Features

- Akathisia is a subjective feeling of restlessness described by patients as a constant need to move.
- Patients pace, make rocking motions while sitting, and frequently change positions.
- The appearance of akathisia is often confused with psychotic agitation or anxiety.

Epidemiology

- Akathisia occurs with dopamine receptor antagonists.
- It is most common in **middle-aged women.**
- It usually occurs within the **first few weeks** of therapy or **after dose changes.**
- Akathisia has also been associated with selective serotonin reuptake inhibitors.

Etiology

- Akathisia *may* be due to an imbalance between noradrenergic and dopaminergic systems.

Treatment

- Akathisia is often difficult to treat.
- The first-line medication is propranolol (beta-adrenergic antagonist).
- Anticholinergics and benzodiazepines may also be helpful.
- Akathisia is significantly less common with serotonin-dopamine antagonists.

TARDIVE DYSKINESIA (TD)

Clinical Features

- TD is characterized by abnormal, involuntary movements of the mouth, face, limbs, and trunk.
- TD most often affects the mouth with lip smacking, lip puckering, tongue protrusion, and chewing.
- Facial involvement includes grimacing, blinking, and eyebrow/forehead movements.
- Limb and trunk movement is generally described as choreoathetoid.
- Chorea is spasmodic movement that is involuntary, rapid, and irregular.
- Athetoid movements are also involuntary, but slow and serpentine.

Epidemiology

- TD occurs most frequently in **elderly women** (>50 years old).
- It is usually seen after **long-term treatment** (tardive) with dopamine receptor antagonists.
- The risk of developing TD is approximately 4 percent per year.
- The risk of TD is increased in older patients with cognitive and mood disorders.

Tardive Dyskinesia (TD) (continued)

Etiology

- Prolonged dopamine antagonism causes receptors to develop an increased sensitivity to dopamine.

Treatment

- There is no effective treatment for TD.
- Dose reduction or switching the patient to a serotonin-dopamine antagonist may alleviate symptoms.
- TD may occur with serotonin-dopamine antagonists but it is extremely uncommon.
- TD remits spontaneously in some patients (5–40 percent).
- The majority of patients suffer chronically even after the antipsychotic has been discontinued.
- Administer the Abnormal Involuntary Movement Scale (AIMS) every 3–6 months for early detection.

Antidepressants: The Basics

IDENTIFICATION

Tricyclic and Tetracyclic Antidepressants (TCAs)
Amitriptyline (Elavil)
Doxepin (Sinequan)
Imipramine (Tofranil)
Clomipramine (Anafranil)
Desipramine (Norpramin)
Nortriptyline (Pamelor)
Maprotiline (Ludiomil)

Monoamine Oxidase Inhibitors (MAOIs)
Isocarboxazid (Marplan)
Phenelzine (Nardil)
Tranylcypromine (Parnate)

Selective Serotonin Reuptake Inhibitors (SSRIs)
Fluoxetine (Prozac)
Paroxetine (Paxil)
Sertraline (Zoloft)
Fluvoxamine (Luvox)
Citalopram (Celexa)

Novel Antidepressants
Bupropion (Wellbutrin)
Nefazodone (Serzone)
Mirtazapine (Remeron)
Venlafaxine (Effexor)
Trazodone (Desyrel)

CHARACTERISTICS

TCAs block the presynaptic reuptake pumps for norepinephrine and serotonin and allow the neurotransmitters to remain longer at the postsynaptic receptor site. They are effective antidepressants but many patients experience **orthostatic hypotension** and **anticholinergic side effects.**

MAOIs inhibit the monoamine oxidase enzyme from degrading norepinephrine, serotonin, and dopamine in the presynaptic nerve terminal. They are also effective antidepressants, but the risk of a hypertensive crisis and the necessity for a restricted diet without tyramine-containing foods may make MAOIs difficult to tolerate.

SSRIs act specifically on serotonin to inhibit its reuptake at the presynaptic nerve terminal. SSRIs are currently the most widely prescribed antidepressants. They have fewer side effects than TCAs or MAOIs because of more selective action on the serotonergic system. Patients are more likely to complain of nausea and sexual dysfunction with the SSRIs.

Novel antidepressants are structurally distinct from the other 3 classes of antidepressants. They are also indicated for depressive disorders but each has its own mechanism of action and side-effect profile. Bupropion, for example, is an effective antidepressant without the sexual side effects of the SSRIs and venlafaxine has shown some efficacy in *severely* depressed and treatment-refractory patients.

Antidepressants: Depth and Detail

REVIEW

The Amine Hypothesis is the prevailing model in the pathogenesis of depression and is used to govern pharmacologic treatment. The Amine Hypothesis states that depleted stores of amine neurotransmitters are associated with depression. The biological amines are dopamine, norepinephrine, and serotonin. TCAs inhibit the reuptake of serotonin and norepinephrine, MAOIs inhibit the degradation of all 3 amines, and SSRIs selectively inhibit the serotonin reuptake pump. All of the antidepressants have comparable clinical efficacy, but SSRIs are associated with fewer side effects and significantly less danger in overdose. SSRIs are widely prescribed today, and it is important to know the differences between them, and when to choose a particular one. The major differences among the SSRIs lies in their pharmacokinetic profiles. There is also a newer group of antidepressants that have combined effects on amine availability and vary in their receptor selectivity and side-effect profiles. The novel antidepressants are gaining popularity because of good clinical efficacy and potentially fewer side effects. This section will review the mechanism of action, indications, side effects, pharmacokinetics, dosage and administration, and precautions of the different classes of antidepressants.

TRICYCLIC AND TETRACYCLIC ANTIDEPRESSANTS (TCAS)

Mechanism of Action
- TCAs increase the availability of norepinephrine *and* serotonin by blockade of *presynaptic* reuptake pumps.

Indications
- **Depressive disorders**
- **Panic disorder**
- **Enuresis** (imipramine)
- **Obsessive-compulsive disorder** (clomipramine)
- **Chronic pain,** including migraine headache and neuropathy (amitriptyline)
- **Bulimia nervosa**

Side Effects
- **Orthostatic hypotension** due to alpha-1 adrenergic blockade is the most *common* side effect of TCAs.
- **Cardiac toxicity** with slowed conduction (e.g., prolonged QT) is the most *severe* adverse effect.
- **Sedation** due to histaminergic blockade.
- **Tremor** and **insomnia** because of increased sympathomimetic activity.
- **Blurred vision, constipation,** and **confusion** due to anticholinergic effects.
- Overdose with TCAs can be fatal due to cardiac arrhythmias, respiratory depression, or coma.

Pharmacokinetics
- TCAs have half-lives that vary from 10 to 70 hours.

Tricyclic and Tetracyclic Antidepressants (TCAS) (continued)

Dosage and Administration

- Antidepressant effects take 2–4 weeks to appear.
- The choice of TCA depends on individual pharmacokinetics and side-effect profiles.
- A baseline EKG should be administered before initiating treatment.
- Routine EKG monitoring is necessary in children.
- When discontinuing treatment a slow taper is required to avoid cholinergic rebound.

Precautions

- TCAs are contraindicated during **pregnancy** and **breast-feeding.**
- **MAOIs** can cause hypertensive crisis *or* serotonin syndrome if co-administered with TCAs.
- Serotonin syndrome may occur with concomitant used of **SSRIs.**
- TCAs should not be used in patients with cardiac arrhythmias (e.g., BBB or prolonged QT).

MONOAMINE OXIDASE INHIBITORS (MAOIS)

Mechanism of Action

- MAOIs *irreversibly* inhibit the metabolism of the biogenic amines in the presynaptic nerve terminal.
- MAO_A is the enzyme responsible for the degradation of serotonin, norepinephrine, and dopamine.
- MAO_B is specific for dopamine metabolism.
- Selegiline is a selective MAO_B inhibitor used for the treatment of Parkinson's disease.

Indications

- **Depression,** particularly **atypical depression**
- **Panic disorder**

Side Effects

- **Insomnia** and **orthostatic hypotension** are the most common side effects.
- **Hepatotoxicity** with phenelzine and tranylcypromine.
- **Hypertensive crisis** may occur with tyramine-containing foods such as beer, cheese, or wine.
- The prodromal symptoms of hypertensive crisis are headache, nausea, vomiting, and sweating.
- Hypertensive crisis may result in cardiac arrhythmias, myocardial infarction, stroke, coma, and death and should be treated immediately with phentolamine (alpha-adrenergic antagonist).

Pharmacokinetics

- MAOIs have short half-lives of approximately 3 hours.

Dosage and Administration

- Antidepressant effects occur within 2–4 weeks.
- Liver function tests should be monitored periodically because of the risk of hepatotoxicity.

Precautions

- **Tyramine**-containing foods are contraindicated (e.g., beer, red wine, cheese, cured meats or fish).
- Patients must allow at least 2 weeks after the last dose of an MAOI before ingesting tyramine.
- Many medications are contraindicated with MAOIs: **SSRIs** and **TCAs** because of serotonin syndrome; **opioids** because of autonomic instability and delirium; **sympathomimetics** because of hypertensive crisis; and **antihypertensives** because of hypotension.

SELECTIVE SEROTONIN REUPTAKE INHIBITORS (SSRIS)

Mechanism of Action
- SSRIs increase the availability of serotonin by inhibiting the *presynaptic* reuptake pump.

Indications
- **Depressive disorders**
- **Anxiety disorders** (especially panic disorder and obsessive-compulsive disorder)
- **Bulimia nervosa** (fluoxetine)
- Other indications include premenstrual dysphoric disorder, migraine headaches, impulsivity, and affective instability in personality disorders.

Side Effects
- The majority of patients treated with SSRIs experience only mild side effects.
- If side effects do occur, it is usually within the first 2 weeks of treatment.
- The most common side effects are **nausea** and **diarrhea** and they occur most often with sertraline.
- **Sedation** is most frequently seen with paroxetine and fluvoxamine.
- **Headache, anxiety** and **insomnia** are most likely to occur with fluoxetine.
- **Sexual dysfunction** may include decreased libido, anorgasmia, or delayed ejaculation and can occur with all the SSRIs.
- **Weight gain** may be seen with paroxetine, sertraline, or fluvoxamine.
- **Serotonin syndrome** is a potentially fatal complication that occurs with serotonin overload.
- Serotonin syndrome is characterized by (1) **autonomic instability** (tachycardia, hypertension, diaphoresis, and hyperpyrexia), (2) **motor problems** (shivering, myoclonus, tremor, and hyperreflexia), and (3) **behavioral disturbances** (agitation, restlessness, delirium, and coma).
- Serotonin syndrome may appear similar to neuroleptic malignant syndrome, but does *not* include rigidity and dystonic reactions (see "Extrapyramidal Symptoms" chapter).
- **SSRI discontinuation syndrome** is a complication of abrupt withdrawal from treatment.
- Paroxetine is the SSRI most likely to cause a discontinuation syndrome because of its short half-life.
- The somatic symptoms of withdrawal include dizziness, nausea, fatigue, myalgia, and insomnia.
- The psychiatric symptoms of withdrawal include anxiety, agitation, irritability, depressed or labile mood, crying spells, impaired concentration, and memory problems.

Pharmacokinetics
- Fluvoxamine has the shortest half-life (15hrs) and fluoxetine has the longest (2–3days).
- Fluoxetine is the only SSRI with an active metabolite (norfluoxetine).
- Paroxetine and citalopram have half-lives that are *increased* in the elderly, so dose reductions are necessary in this population.
- Paroxetine is the most potent SSRI and fluvoxamine is the least.
- All SSRIs are metabolized by the liver but only fluoxetine requires dose reductions with liver disease.
- Fluvoxamine is a good choice for patients on multiple drug therapy because its short half-life minimizes the risk of drug-drug interactions.

Selective Serotonin Reuptake Inhibitors (SSRIS) (continued)

Dosage and Administration

- The antidepressant effect of SSRIs usually takes 2 to 4 weeks to appear.
- SSRIs are generally effective for depression at the lower end of the dose range.
- Higher doses tend to increase the risk of adverse events *without* increasing antidepressant activity.
- Physicians should wait at least **4** weeks before evaluating the *antidepressant* activity of an SSRI.
- In obsessive-compulsive disorder, **6 to 8** weeks are required before evaluating SSRI effectiveness.
- Obsessive-compulsive disorder usually requires higher doses of SSRIs than depression.
- Fluoxetine should be administered in an alternate-day regimen to patients with renal impairment.
- Fluoxetine is administered in the morning to avoid insomnia because it is the most activating SSRI.
- Paroxetine is usually given in the evening because it is the most sedating SSRI.
- Sertraline can be taken with meals to reduce nausea because it is the most likely to cause GI distress.
- SSRI treatment of depression should continue for 6 months after response has been obtained.
- Patients with a history of recurrent disease should continue treatment for 18 months after response.
- SSRIs should be tapered slowly to avoid SSRI discontinuation syndrome.

Precautions

- **MAOIs** are contraindicated because of serotonin syndrome and a **2**-week wash-out period is necessary before starting an MAOI after SSRI treatment.
- A **5**-week out wash-out period is necessary with fluoxetine because of its long elimination half-life.
- Caution must be exercised in using SSRIs during pregnancy and breast-feeding.
- Fluvoxamine is contraindicated with terfenadine, astemizole, and cisapride because it inhibits the liver enzyme (CYP450 3A4) responsible for their metabolism.

Table: Distinguishing Characteristics of SSRIs

Medication	Half-Life	Dose Range	Side Effects
Fluvoxamine (Luvox)	15 hours	100–300 mg/day	Nausea Ejaculatory delay
Paroxetine (Paxil)	21 hours	20–60 mg/day	Sedation Nausea
Sertraline (Zoloft)	25 hours	50–200 mg/day	Nausea Ejaculatory delay
Citalopram (Celexa)	33 hours	20–60 mg/day	Nausea Sedation
Fluoxetine (Prozac)	2–3 **days**	20–80 mg/day	Insomnia Nausea

BUPROPION (WELLBUTRIN)

Mechanism of Action
- Bupropion is a norepinephrine and dopamine reuptake inhibitor.

Indications
- **Depressive disorders**
- **Smoking cessation** (the brand name is Zyban)
- Adjunctive treatment for **ADHD**

Side Effects
- **Agitation, dry mouth, insomnia,** and **nausea** are the most frequent side effects.
- There is an increased risk of **seizures** at high doses (>450 mg).
- Bupropion may aggravate psychotic symptoms.
- There are significantly fewer sexual side effects as compared to the SSRIs.
- There is **no** orthostatic hypotension, weight gain, or sedation.

Pharmacokinetics
- The half-life of bupropion varies from 8 to 40 hours.

Dosage and Administration
- Antidepressant effects of bupropion occur 2 to 4 weeks after the initial dose.

Precautions
- Patients with a history of **head trauma, brain tumor,** or **seizure disorder** should not take bupropion because it may reduce the seizure threshold.
- Patients with **anorexia nervosa** and **bulimia nervosa** may also have an increased risk of seizures.
- Women who are **pregnant** or **nursing** should not take bupropion.
- The combination of bupropion and **MAOIs** can induce serotonin syndrome.

NEFAZODONE (SERZONE)

Mechanism of Action
- Nefazadone has the combined effects of selective serotonin reuptake inhibition and 5-HT$_2$ **antagonism.**
- The dual action may selectively activate **5-HT$_1$ receptors to specifically reduce depression and anxiety.**
- Nefazodone also has properties of norepinephrine reuptake inhibition.

Indications
- **Depressive disorders**
- **Panic disorder**
- **Posttraumatic stress disorder**

Side Effects
- **Sedation, nausea,** and **dry mouth.**
- Alpha-1 antagonism may cause **orthostatic hypotension, dizziness,** and **headache.**
- Nefazodone does *not* cause sexual dysfunction or weight gain.

Nefazodone (Serzone) (continued)

Pharmacokinetics
- Nefazodone has a half-life of approximately 5 hours.

Dosage and Administration
- Antidepressant effects occur within 2 to 4 weeks.

Precautions
- Nefazodone inhibits the liver enzyme (CYP450 3A4) that metabolizes **triazolam** (Halcion), **alprazolam** (Xanax), terfenadine, astemizole, cisapride, pimozide, and carbamazepine and must be used carefully with these medications.
- It is not recommended for use in **pregnant** or **nursing women.**
- **MAOIs** may induce serotonin syndrome if co-administered with nefazodone.

VENLAFAXINE (EFFEXOR)

Mechanism of Action
- Venlafaxine is a non-selective inhibitor of amine reuptake (serotonin, norepinephrine, and dopamine).
- It does *not* affect cholinergic, histaminergic, or adrenergic receptors.

Indications
- **Depressive disorders**
- Venlafaxine may be particularly effective for severely depressed patients.
- Patients previously refractory to antidepressant treatment may respond to venlafaxine.
- Anxiety disorders (specifically **generalized anxiety disorder, PTSD, panic disorder,** and **OCD**)

Side Effects
- **Sedation, nausea, dizziness,** and **nervousness,** are the most common side effects.
- **Increased blood pressure** may occur in some patients and BP should be monitored.
- **Ejaculatory delay** may occur in males.
- Abrupt withdrawal may produce a **discontinuation syndrome** (e.g., insomnia and nausea).

Pharmacokinetics
- The half-life of venlafaxine is approximately 5 hours.

Dosage and Administration
- The antidepressant effects of venlafaxine may appear earlier than with other antidepressants.
- A slow taper over at least 1-week is required to avoid a discontinuation syndrome.
- Routine monitoring of blood pressure may be necessary.

Precautions
- Venlafaxine is not recommended in **pregnant** and **nursing women.**
- **MAOIs** are contraindicated because of serotonin syndrome.
- It must be used cautiously in patients with preexisting hypertension.

MIRTAZAPINE (REMERON)

Mechanism of Action
- Mirtazapine is an alpha-2 antagonist, a 5-HT$_2$ antagonist, and a 5-HT$_3$ antagonist.
- The dual antagonism of type 2 and 3 serotonin receptors causes a net *activation* of 5-HT$_1$ receptors.
- The cumulative effect of mirtazapine is to increase adrenergic and serotonergic activity.
- It is known as a noradrenergic and specific serotonergic antidepressant (NaSSA).

Indications
- **Depressive disorders**
- **Anxiety disorders**
- **Insomnia**

Side Effects
- **Sedation** is the most common side effect because of potent antihistaminergic properties.
- Most patients will experience *less* sedation at higher doses of mirtazapine ($\geq$30 mg).
- **Increased appetite, weight gain** and **dizziness** are also frequent side effects.
- **Dry mouth** and **constipation** occur because mirtazapine has anticholinergic activity.
- Mirtazapine (like buproprion and nefazodone) has significantly fewer sexual side effects than SSRIs.

Pharmacokinetics
- The half-life of mirtazapine is 20–40 hours.

Dosage and Administration
- Antidepressant effects occur after 2 to 4 weeks, but may appear within 1 week of treatment.

Precautions
- Mirtazapine should be discontinued if the patient has a **low WBC** or shows signs of **infection** because there have been isolated reports of neutropenia.
- **Pregnant** and **nursing** women should not take mirtazapine.
- **MAOIs** may induce serotonin syndrome.

TRAZODONE (DESYREL)

Mechanism of Action
- Trazodone is structurally related to alprazolam (Xanax), a benzodiazepine with antidepressant activity.
- It acts by specific presynaptic serotonin reuptake inhibition and postsynaptic 5-HT$_2$ *antagonism*.
- Trazodone also has properties of alpha-1 adrenergic and histaminergic antagonism.

Indications
- **Depressive disorders**
- **Insomnia**
- **Anxiety disorders**

Trazodone (Desyrel) (continued)

Side Effects

- **Orthostatic hypotension** and **dizziness** (alpha-1 blockade) are the most common side effects.
- **Sedation** (antihistaminergic activity) is also frequent and the reason for its effectiveness as a hypnotic.
- **Priapism** is a rare but potentially dangerous side effect that can lead to impotence.
- Headache and GI distress are other possible side effects.

Pharmacokinetics

- Trazodone has a half-life of 3–9 hours.

Dosage and Administration

- Antidepressant effects take 2 to 4 weeks to appear.
- Sedative effects occur within 1 hour.
- A slow upward titration is required to avoid orthostatic hypotension and possibly falls in the elderly.

Precautions

- Trazodone should not be given with **antihypertensive medications.**
- It is not recommended for use with **electroconvulsive treatment.**
- Trazodone is contraindicated in women who are **pregnant** or **nursing.**
- **MAOIs** increase the risk of developing serotonin syndrome.

Table: Distinguishing Characteristics of the Novel Antidepressants

Medication	Mechanism of Action	Side Effects
Bupropion (Wellbutrin)	NE & DA reuptake inhibitor	Agitation Nausea Increased risk of seizures
Nefazodone (Serzone)	5-HT & NE reuptake inhibitor 5-HT$_{2A}$ antagonist	Sedation Nausea Orthostatic hypotension
Venlafaxine (Effexor)	Non-selective (5-HT,NE, & DA) reuptake inhibitor	Sedation Nausea Elevated blood pressure
Mirtazapine (Remeron)	NaSSA (noradrenergic and selective serotonin agonist) Alpha-2 antagonist 5-HT$_{2/3}$ antagonist	Sedation (initially) Weight gain Dry mouth and constipation
Trazodone (Desyrel)	5-HT reuptake inhibitor 5-HT$_{2A}$ antagonist alpha-1 antagonist	Sedation Orthostatic hypotension Priapism

IDENTIFICATION

Anxiolytics can be divided into 2 categories: benzodiazepines and non-benzodiazepines.

Benzodiazepines

Diazepam (Valium)

Clonazepam (Klonopin)

Alprazolam (Xanax)

Lorazepam (Ativan)

Chlordiazepoxide (Librium)

Temazepam (Restoril)

Triazolam (Halcion)

Flurazepam (Dalmane)

Midazolam (Versed)

Non-Benzodiazepines

Buspirone (BuSpar)

Zolpidem (Ambien)

CHARACTERISTICS

Benzodiazepines bind to the $GABA_A$ receptor complex and increase the activity of gamma-aminobutyric acid (GABA), an *inhibitory* neurotransmitter. Benzodiazepines are mainly used to treat anxiety and insomnia. They are also effective as anticonvulsants and muscle relaxants.

Non-Benzodiazepines are buspirone and zolpidem. Buspirone is a serotonin 1A receptor agonist used for generalized anxiety disorder. Zolpidem is a *non*-benzodiazepine that acts on the benzodiazepine receptor complex to increase GABA. Zolpidem is used only for the treatment of insomnia and does *not* have anxiolytic, anticonvulsant, or muscle relaxant properties.

Anxiolytics: Depth and Detail

REVIEW

Benzodiazepines are GABA agonists that are widely prescribed for the treatment of anxiety and insomnia. The choice of benzodiazepine depends on differences in their onset of action, half-lives, and potency. Benzodiazepines that have a rapid onset of action due to high lipid solubility (diazepam, clonazepam, flurazepam, and triazolam) can produce a euphoric feeling and increase the risk of abuse and dependence. Rapid onset of action refers to the rate of *absorption* and is not the same as "short-acting." Short-acting refers to the average half-life of metabolites and the rate of *elimination*. Short-acting benzodiazepines may have rapid *or* slow rates of absorption and are used for insomnia to avoid residual daytime drowsiness (triazolam, lorazepam, temazepam, and alprazolam). Long-acting benzodiazepines are more suitable for generalized anxiety disorder. Buspirone is a non-benzodiazepine anxiolytic agent *without* sedative effects or abuse potential. It is frequently used to treat anxiety in patients with a history of substance abuse. Zolpidem is a non-benzodiazepine that is specifically indicated for the treatment of insomnia. This section will review the mechanism of action, indications, side effects, pharmacokinetics, dosage and administration, and precautions of benzodiazepines and non-benzodiazepines.

BENZODIAZEPINES

Mechanism of Action
- Benzodiazepines enhance the activity of GABA by binding to the GABA$_A$ receptor complex.
- They are direct agonists of GABA function and their effect is almost immediate.

Indications
- **Generalized anxiety disorder**
- **Adjustment disorder with anxiety**
- **Insomnia** (short-acting benzodiazepines—triazolam, lorazepam, temazepam, and alprazolam)
- **Panic disorder** and **social phobia** (alprazolam and clonazepam)
- **Obsessive-compulsive disorder** (clonazepam)
- **Acute mania** (clonazepam)
- **Alcohol withdrawal** (chlordiazepoxide and lorazepam)
- **Acute agitation** (Lorazepam IM/PO)
- **Hyperarousal** in posttraumatic stress disorder
- *Acute* **treatment of seizures** (lorazepam and diazepam)
- **Medical procedures** (e.g., colonoscopy–midazolam has profound sedative and amnestic effects)

Benzodiazepines (continued)

Side Effects

- **Drowsiness** is the most common side effect.
- **Dizziness** occurs less frequently.
- **Anterograde amnesia** may be seen with high-potency benzodiazepines (triazolam, alprazolam, clonazepam, lorazepam, and midazolam).
- A **withdrawal syndrome** can occur with abrupt termination of benzodiazepines.
- Withdrawal symptoms include depression, anxiety, insomnia, irritability, and **seizures.**
- **Tolerance** and **dependence** may develop with prolonged use of benzodiazepines.
- **Respiratory depression** may occur when benzodiazepines are combined with other sedatives (e.g., alcohol).
- Signs of intoxication are **confusion, slurred speech, ataxia,** and **hyporeflexia.**
- Benzodiazepines are safe in *overdose* unless combined with other drugs (e.g., alcohol, antipsychotics, and antidepressants) to cause **respiratory depression, coma,** and **death.**

Pharmacokinetics

- Long-acting benzodiazepines (diazepam, flurazepam, and chlordiazepoxide) have half-lives of approximately 100 hours.
- Clonazepam is also considered a long-acting benzodiazepine, but its half-life is less than 50 hours.
- Short-acting agents (alprazolam, lorazepam, midazolam, temazepam, and triazolam) have half-lives of between 2–20 hours.
- Triazolam (Halcion) is the shortest acting of all the benzodiazepines with a half-life of 2–3 hours.

Dosage and Administration

- Anxiolytic and sedative effects of benzodiazepines occur within 30–60 minutes.
- Benzodiazepines should be administered only for relatively short periods of time.
- Greater than 6 weeks of benzodiazepine use increases the risk of tolerance, dependence, and withdrawal syndromes.
- A gradual taper of 15 to 25 *percent* per week is usually sufficient to avoid withdrawal symptoms.
- High doses of short-acting benzodiazepines increase the risk of withdrawal symptoms.
- Alprazolam is a high-potency, short-acting ($t\frac{1}{2}$ = 12hrs) benzodiazepine that is most frequently associated with symptoms of withdrawal.
- Benzodiazepines need to be used carefully in elderly patients for fear of falls from sedation.

Precautions

- Benzodiazepines should be avoided in patients with pre-existing **cognitive impairment** and **delirium.**
- They should also be avoided in patients with **lung disease** (including obstructive sleep apnea) because of increased risk of respiratory depression.
- Benzodiazepines should not be used with other **CNS depressants** (e.g., alcohol, barbiturates, opioids).
- Benzodiazepine use during **pregnancy** can cause a withdrawal syndrome in neonates.
- Secretion in breast milk may affect nursing babies (e.g., drowsiness and dyspnea).

Benzodiazepines (continued)

Table: Distinguishing Characteristics of Benzodiazepines

Drug	Duration(Acting)	Half-Life(hours)	Onset of Action
Alprazolam (Xanax)	Short	12	Medium
Lorazepam (Ativan)	Short	15	Medium
Triazolam (Halcion)	Short	2	Fast
Temazepam (Restoril)	Short	11	Medium
Midazolam (Versed)	Short	2.5	Fast (IV only)
Diazepam (Valium)	Long	100	Fast
Clonazepam (Klonopin)	Long	34	Fast
Flurazepam (Dalmane)	Long	100	Fast
Chlordiazepoxide (Librium)	Long	100	Medium

Adapted from Kaplan HI, Sadock VA: Kaplan and Sadock's Synopsis of Psychiatry, 8th ed. Baltimore, Lippincott Williams & Wilkins, 1997.

BUSPIRONE (BUSPAR)

Mechanism of Action
- Buspirone is a serotonin 1A (5-HT$_{1A}$) receptor agonist.
- 5-HT$_{1A}$ receptors are inhibitory and buspirone may *decrease* serotonergic release.
- The precise effect on symptoms of anxiety is unclear.

Indications
- **Generalized anxiety disorder**
- **Anxiety** in patients with a **history of substance abuse** because it does *not* have abuse potential.
- Adjunctive treatment of **obsessive-compulsive disorder** and **depression.**
- Buspirone does *not* have sedating, anticonvulsant, or muscle relaxing effects like benzodiazepines.

Side Effects
- The most frequent side effects are **headache, dizziness, restlessness,** and **nausea.**
- There is *no* withdrawal syndrome associated with buspirone.

Pharmacokinetics
- The half-life of buspirone is 2–11 hours.

Dosage and Administration
- The therapeutic effect on anxiety may take 2–3 weeks to occur.
- Buspirone treatment may temporarily require benzodiazepines until full effect is reached (2–3 wks).
- Because of its short half-life, three times daily dosing is required.

Precautions
- Buspirone is contraindicated with **MAOIs** because of the risk of serotonin syndrome (see "Antidepressants" chapter).
- It should be used with caution during pregnancy and breast-feeding.

ZOLPIDEM (AMBIEN)

Mechanism of Action
- Zolpidem is a non-benzodiazepine gamma-aminobutyric acid (GABA) agonist.
- It binds to the same receptor complex as benzodiazepines (GABA$_A$).

Indications
- Zolpidem is indicated for the treatment of **insomnia.**
- It has *not* been shown to have significant anxiolytic, anticonvulsant, or muscle-relaxant properties.
- Zaleplon is a newer non-benzodiazepine similar to zolpidem that is also used for insomnia.

Side Effects
- **Dizziness, headache, nausea, and vomiting** are the most frequent side effects.
- A **withdrawal syndrome** similar to that seen with benzodiazepines may occur after long-term use.

Pharmacokinetics
- Zolpidem is very short-acting with a half-life of 2–3 hours.

Dosage and Administration
- Sedative effects usually occur within 30 minutes.
- A dose of 10 mg at night is usually sufficient to induce sleep in adults.
- Elderly patients should start with 5 mg at night.

Precautions
- Zolpidem is secreted in breast milk and not recommended during breast-feeding.

IDENTIFICATION

There are 3 mood stabilizers that are most commonly used:

1) Lithium carbonate (Eskalith, Eskalith CR, Lithobid, Lithonate)

2) Valproic acid (Depakene) and divalproex sodium (Depakote)

3) Carbamazepine (Tegretol)

CHARACTERISTICS

The mood stabilizers are used mainly for bipolar disorder. They are also frequently used for mood instability and impulsivity.

Lithium carbonate is the classic mood stabilizer and until recently was the first-line treatment for bipolar disorder.

Valproic acid is an anticonvulsant that many psychiatrists are now using as the first-line treatment for bipolar disorder. It has fewer side effects than lithium for some patients and has been shown to be more effective in rapid cycling and mixed episodes of bipolar disorder.

Carbamazepine is an anticonvulsant that is generally used as a second-line agent in the treatment of bipolar disorder. It may also be more effective than lithium in treating rapid cycling and mixed episode types of bipolar disorder.

Mood Stabilizers: Depth and Detail

REVIEW

Lithium is the classic mood stabilizer and was first used for bipolar disorder in 1949. Recently, some psychiatrists have replaced lithium with valproic acid because of a significantly reduced side-effect profile. Anticonvulsant medications in general are gaining popularity in treating bipolar disorder. In addition to valproic acid and carbamazepine, **gabapentin (Neurontin)** and **lamotrigine (Lamictal)** are two more anticonvulsants that are being used with increasing frequency as *second-line* treatments, and controlled studies are underway. This section will review the mechanism of action, indications, side effects, pharmacokinetics, dosage and administration, and precautions of the most commonly used mood stabilizers.

LITHIUM CARBONATE

Mechanism of Action
* The mechanism of action of lithium is unclear.
* One theory is that lithium acts by blocking inositol phosphatases,
* The inhibition of inositol phosphate metabolism decreases the action of neurotransmitters linked to this second messenger system (e.g., serotonin and norepinephrine)

Indications
* **Acute mania** associated with bipolar I and schizoaffective disorder
* Lithium *maintenance* to prevent relapse in **bipolar I disorder**
* *Adjunctive* treatment in **major depression** not responsive to antidepressants alone
* **Impulsivity** and **affective instability** associated with personality disorders

Side Effects
* The most common side effects of lithium treatment are gastrointestinal distress, weight gain, fine tremor, and cognitive impairment.
* **Weight gain** is a frequent complaint and patients need to exercise and maintain a normal diet.
* **Fine tremor** usually involves the hands and fingers and may be treated with propranolol.
* **Cognitive impairment** is described as "clouding," with memory and concentration difficulties.
* Lithium is an antagonist to antidiuretic hormone and may cause **polyuria** and secondary polydipsia.
* It may impair thyroid function and result in **hypothyroidism.**
* It displaces intracellular potassium and causes **hypokalemia** with flattened T waves on EKG.
* At *toxic* levels lithium can induce ataxia, coarse tremor, seizures, and coma.

Pharmacokinetics
* The half-life of lithium is approximately 20 hours.
* Steady state is reached after **5 days** and serum levels should be between **0.6 and 1.2 mEq/L** for *maintenance* treatment and between **1.0 and 1.5 mEq/L** for *acute* treatment.
* It is eliminated mainly by the kidneys.
* Kidney function must be evaluated before administering lithium, particularly in the elderly.
* Diuretics, NSAIDs, and ACE inhibitors increase lithium levels.

Lithium Carbonate (continued)

Dosage and Administration
- The therapeutic response of lithium should occur within 1 to 3 weeks.
- Serum levels should be measured after **5 days** at any given dosage.
- Monitor serum levels weekly for 2 months and then biweekly for another 2 months.

Precautions
- Lithium use during the first trimester of **pregnancy** increases the risk of congenital anomalies.
- The most common congenital defect is Ebstein's anomaly of the tricuspid valve.
- Patients should not **breast-feed** because lithium is excreted in breast milk.
- Lithium is contraindicated in **renal insufficiency** because it is cleared by the kidneys.

VALPROIC ACID

Mechanism of Action
- Valproic acid is a GABA agonist that decreases neuronal excitability.
- The precise effect of valproic acid on psychiatric illness is unclear.
- Valproic acid is the active compound that gets converted from sodium valproate in the stomach.

Indications
- **Acute mania** in bipolar I disorder and schizoaffective disorder
- It is more effective than lithium in treating **rapid cycling** and **mixed episodes** of bipolar disorder.
- Maintenance treatment may prevent relapse in **bipolar I disorder**
- Augmentation of antipsychotic medication in the treatment of **schizophrenia**
- **Impulsivity** and **affective instability** associated with personality disorders.
- *Generalized* seizures in **epilepsy.**

Side Effects
- The most common side effects of valproic acid are **sedation, dizziness, nausea,** and **weight gain.**
- Gastrointestinal side effects are reduced by using divalproex (Depakote).
- Divalproex is a *sustained* release, enteric-coated preparation.
- The most serious adverse effect is **hepatitis,** and liver function needs to be checked periodically.
- **Pancreatitis** is a rare, but severe side effect.
- Hematological side effects include **thrombocytopenia,** and platelets need to be checked periodically.
- Neurological side effects include tremor, ataxia, dysarthria, and headaches.
- The symptoms of valproic acid *toxicity* are somnolence, heart block, and coma.

Pharmacokinetics
- The half-life of valproic acid is approximately 10 hours.
- It is metabolized by the liver.

Dosage and Administration
- The therapeutic response should occur within 1 to 2 weeks.
- Doses should be reduced in the elderly.
- Serum valproic acid levels should be assessed after **3 days.**
- Symptom relief usually occurs at serum levels between **50–125 μg/ml**.
- Serum levels should be monitored weekly for the first 2 months and then biweekly for 2 months.

Valproic Acid (continued)

Precautions

- Valproic acid is contraindicated in **pregnancy** and **nursing** because it may cause neural tube defects.
- Patients with **hepatic disease** should not use valproic acid.

CARBAMAZEPINE (TEGRETOL)

Mechanism of Action

- Carbamazepine binds to voltage-gated sodium channels and decreases transmission across synapses.
- It was traditionally used as an anticonvulsant, and its effect on psychiatric illness is unclear.

Indications

- **Acute mania** in bipolar I and schizoaffective disorder
- It is more effective than lithium in treating **rapid cycling** and **mixed episodes** of bipolar disorder.
- *Prophylactic* maintenance treatment in **bipolar I disorder**
- Adjunctive treatment in **schizophrenia**
- **Impulsivity** and **affective instability** associated with personality disorders
- Symptom reduction in **benzodiazepine** and **alcohol withdrawal**
- **Epilepsy** and **trigeminal neuralgia.**

Side Effects

- The most common adverse effects of carbamazepine are on the central nervous system and gastrointestinal tract.
- **Central nervous system** side effects include sedation, dizziness, ataxia, and confusion.
- **Gastrointestinal** side effects are nausea, vomiting, diarrhea or constipation, and loss of appetite.
- **Hematological** side effects are rare but may include thrombocytopenia, aplastic anemia, and agranulocytosis.
- **Hepatic** side effects are hepatitis and cholestatic jaundice.
- **Dermatological** effects are relatively common and may include rash, urticaria, or rarely Stevens-Johnson syndrome.
- **Cardiac** side effects are rare, but may include decreased conduction and congestive heart failure.
- Signs of toxicity are confusion, stupor, tachycardia, seizures, respiratory depression, and coma.

Pharmacokinetics

- The half-life of carbamazepine is highly variable
- It is absorbed erratically from the gastrointestinal tract but food facilitates absorption.
- After long-term administration the half-life is approximately 15 hours.
- Carbamazepine is metabolized by the liver and cleared by the kidneys.
- Because of induction of hepatic microsomal enzymes such as P450, carbamazepine may interact significantly with many other drugs by increasing or decreasing their metabolism.
- Carbamazepine may decrease the effectiveness of oral contraceptive pills and antipsychotics.

Carbamazepine (Tegretol) (continued)

Dosage and Administration

- The mood stabilizing effects occur within 1 to 2 weeks.
- Doses should be reduced in the elderly.
- Upward titration must be done carefully and should not exceed 200 mg/day.
- Complete blood count should be checked periodically to assess hematological side effects (thrombocytopenia, aplastic anemia, and agranulocytosis).
- Serum carbamazepine levels should be assessed after **5 days** at any given dosage.
- Serum levels of **8–12 µg/ml** should be achieved.
- Levels should be measured weekly for 2 months and then biweekly for another 2 months.

Precautions

- Carbamazepine is not recommended during **pregnancy** and **breast-feeding.**
- During pregnancy there is an increased risk of congenital malformations such as spina bifida.
- **Hepatic disease, hematological disease,** and **cardiac disease** are all *relative* contraindications.

Other Treatments: The Basics

IDENTIFICATION

1) Psychostimulants
   a) Methylphenidate (Ritalin)
   b) Dextroamphetamine (Dexedrine)
   c) Amphetamine/dextroamphetamine (Adderall)
   d) Pemoline (Cylert)

2) Clonidine (Catapres)

3) Beta-Blockers
   a) Propranolol (Inderal)

4) Anticholinergics
   a) Benztropine (Cogentin)
   b) Trihexyphenidyl (Artane)

5) Electroconvulsive Therapy (ECT)

6) Thyroid Hormone
   a) Liothyronine (Cytomel)
   b) Levothyroxine (Synthroid)

CHARACTERISTICS

Psychostimulants are sympathomimetic medications that increase the release of norepinephrine, dopamine, and serotonin. They are used to treat attention deficit in children (methylphenidate), narcolepsy (pemoline), or as adjunctive treatment in depression (dextroamphetamine).

Clonidine is an alpha 2-receptor agonist that *decreases* the release of sympathetic neurotransmitters. It is traditionally used to treat hypertension, but in psychiatric settings it is helpful for the symptoms of opioid withdrawal, Tourette's disorder, and hyperactivity and aggression in children.

Beta-Blockers also decrease sympathetic discharge by inhibiting beta-adrenergic receptors. They are effective in treating the peripheral symptoms of anxiety because they reduce sweating, tachycardia, palpitations, and tremors. Beta-blockers are also the first-line treatment for acute akathisia.

Anticholinergics act as antagonists at muscarinic acetylcholine receptors. They are used in psychiatry to treat extrapyramidal symptoms associated with antipsychotic treatment. Anticholinergic medication is particularly effective for antipsychotic-induced parkinsonism, acute dystonia, and postural tremor.

Electroconvulsive Therapy induces seizure-like activity and effectively treats symptoms of depression and mania through a mechanism that is not fully understood. ECT is generally only used after patients fail medication trials or in cases of acute suicidal, homicidal, or psychotic depression.

Thyroid hormone medications are isomers of the hormone itself. They are used as adjuncts in the treatment of depression because of evidence that the hypothalamic/pituitary/adrenal axis is disturbed in depressed patients. Other uses include lithium-induced hypothyroidism and rapid-cycling bipolar disorder.

Other Treatments: Depth and Detail

REVIEW

Many medications that are used in psychiatry have not been traditionally considered psychiatric medications. The list of these medications is rapidly expanding but this section will discuss only those that are most frequently used clinically and asked about on examinations. **Clonidine** and **beta-blockers** have side effects such as sedation and reduced sympathetic tone that are exploited for their potential in psychiatric settings. **Anticholinergic medications** effectively counter the extrapyramidal symptoms associated with antipsychotic dopaminergic blockade. Low levels of **thyroid hormone** have been associated with depressive states, and adding the hormone to antidepressant medications may be useful in treating depression. **Psychostimulants** are sympathomimetic drugs that are used to treat ADHD, narcolepsy, and depression. **Electroconvulsive therapy** induces seizures to treat depression, mania, and psychosis. Psychostimulants and ECT *are* traditionally considered psychiatric treatments. This section will review the mechanism of action, indications, side effects, pharmacokinetics, dosage and administration, and precautions of selected treatments that do not appropriately fall into any other category.

PSYCHOSTIMULANTS

Mechanism of Action

- Psychostimulants are adrenergic agonists that stimulate the release of catecholamines.
- Methylphenidate (Ritalin) and dextroamphetamine (Dexedrine) are chemically related to amphetamines.
- Adderall is a combination of amphetamine and dextroamphetamine.
- Pemoline (Cylert) has a different structure and its pharmacological actions are less well understood.

Indications

- **Attention deficit/hyperactivity disorder**
- **Narcolepsy**
- **Depressive disorders** that are resistant to treatment
- Affective lability, impulsivity, and attention deficit in adults

Side Effects

- **Anxiety, insomnia,** and **headache** are the most common adverse effects.
- **Tolerance** and **dependence** may develop in some patients.
- There is **abuse potential** because of euphoric properties and potentially improved concentration and productivity.
- Tachycardia, increased blood pressure, and palpitations may occur.
- Decreased appetite and weight loss can occur early in treatment before tolerance develops.
- Psychostimulants may induce tics, dyskinesias, or psychotic symptoms in *vulnerable* patients.
- Transient growth suppression may occur in children because of disturbed growth hormone secretion.
- Pemoline may cause hepatotoxicity.

Pharmacokinetics

- Methylphenidate is the most frequently prescribed psychostimulant and its half-life is 1–2 hours.
- Methylphenidate acts within 30 minutes of administration and lasts 3–4 hours, so multiple daily dosing is required.
- Adderall has a longer half-life than methylphenidate (6–10 hours) and therefore requires fewer dosings.

Psychostimulants (continued)

Dosage and Administration

- Antidepressant effects of psychostimulants typically occur within 1 week.
- Blood pressure and cardiac status should be evaluated before initiating treatment with psychostimulants.
- Growth curves should be monitored in children.
- CBC and liver function tests need to be periodically checked.
- Signs of tolerance and dependence must be assessed.

Precautions

- Psychostimulants are contraindicated during **breast-feeding** and **pregnancy.**
- Patients with hypertension, cardiac disease, glaucoma, or hyperthyroidism should not use psychostimulants.
- They should not be administered to **psychotic patients.**
- They are not recommended for patients with a history of **substance abuse.**

CLONIDINE

Mechanism of Action

- Clonidine (Catapres) is an alpha-2 (α_2) adrenergic receptor agonist.
- Alpha-2 is an inhibitory receptor that *decreases* the release of sympathetic neurotransmitters.
- The primary use of clonidine is to reduce blood pressure.
- In psychiatric disorders its effectiveness is due to reduced sympathetic tone and sedative side effects.

Indications

- **Opioid withdrawal**
- **Tourette's disorder**
- **Hyperactivity** (ADHD) and **aggression** in children

Side Effects

- **Sedation, hypotension,** and **dizziness** are the most troublesome side effects.
- Dry mouth, nausea, constipation, and sexual dysfunction may also occur.

Pharmacokinetics

- The half-life of clonidine is approximately 10 hours.

Dosage and Administration

- The sedative effects occur within 1 hour of administration.
- A slow taper is necessary upon discontinuation to avoid rebound hypertension.
- Patients with heart disease need to have cardiac functioning assessed periodically.

Precautions

- Patients taking other **antihypertensives** must be monitored carefully.

BETA-BLOCKERS

Mechanism of Action

- Beta-adrenergic antagonists inhibit the sympathetic nervous system's response to epinephrine and norepinephrine.
- Propranolol (Inderal) is the most frequently prescribed beta-blocker for psychiatric conditions and it non-selectively affects β_1 and β_2 receptors.
- Beta-1 blockade lowers blood pressure, decreases heart rate, and reduces cardiac contraction.
- Beta-2 blockade *prevents* vasodilation and bronchodilation.
- Beta-blockade is effective in treating anxiety because it reduces the peripheral symptoms of tachycardia, sweating, palpitations, and tremor.

Indications

- **Social phobia** (especially performance type)
- **Acute akathisia** (associated with antipsychotic medication and SSRIs)
- **Postural tremor** (typically lithium-induced)
- Other anxiety disorders (panic disorder, posttraumatic disorder, and generalized anxiety disorder)
- Adjuvant treatment of alcohol withdrawal, aggression, and violent behavior

Side Effects

- **Hypotension** and **bradycardia** are the most common side effects of beta-blockers.
- Nausea, vomiting, diarrhea, and sexual dysfunction (impotence) are less frequent.
- Cognitive functioning may be impaired in some people.
- Depression is a *rare* side effect that has been *over*estimated historically.

Pharmacokinetics

- The half-life of most beta-blockers varies from 3 to 8 hours.
- **Propranolol,** pindolol, and labetalol all affect β_1 and β_2 receptors equally (*non-selective*).
- Metoprolol and atenolol are β_1 *selective.*

Dosage and Administration

- The regimen for performance anxiety is propranolol (10–40 mg) 30 minutes before the event.
- A trial administration is recommended to ensure that propranolol is well tolerated.

Precautions

- Beta-blockers are contraindicated in **insulin-dependent diabetes** because they mask the body's normal sympathetic response to hypoglycemia.
- They are contraindicated in patients with **cardiac conduction abnormalities** because of an increased risk of heart block secondary to β_1 mediated negative inotropic effects.
- Non-selective beta-blockers are not recommended with **asthma** because of β_2-mediated bronchoconstriction.

ANTICHOLINERGICS

Mechanism of Action
- The main effect of anticholinergics is blockade of muscarinic acetylcholine receptors.
- Benztropine (Cogentin) and trihexyphenidyl (Artane) are the most commonly prescribed anticholinergics.
- Anticholinergic activity is thought to be protective against extrapyramidal symptoms associated with mid and high-potency antipsychotic treatment.

Indications
- Antipsychotic-induced **acute dystonia**
- Antipsychotic-induced **parkinsonism**
- Medication-induced **postural tremor**

Side Effects
- **Dry mouth, urinary retention,** and **blurred vision** are the most common side effects.
- Sedation, confusion, and weakness may also occur.
- Elderly patients are more likely to experience memory loss and/or anticholinergic-induced delirium.
- Mild euphoria-producing properties increase abuse potential, particularly with trihexyphenidyl.
- Anticholinergic intoxication is characterized by hallucinations, delirium, seizures, coma, and peripheral signs of flushing, hyperthermia, mydriasis, and dry skin.

Pharmacokinetics
- Trihexyphenidyl and benztropine have half-lives between 3 and 6 hours.

Dosage and Administration
- Anticholinergics act within 1 to 3 hours of administration if given orally.
- Benztropine given intramuscularly for *acute* dystonia should act within 30 minutes.
- Parkinsonism is treated with trihexyphenidyl or benztropine orally (1–2 mg bid-qid).
- Benztropine *prophylaxis* is given to patients with a history of acute dystonic reactions or parkinsonism.
- Anticholinergics require a slow taper over at least 2 weeks to avoid rebound cholinergic side effects.

Precautions
- Anticholinergics should be used carefully with **low-potency antipsychotics** and **tricyclic antidepressants** because of additive anticholinergic effects.
- Prostatic hypertrophy, urinary retention, glaucoma, and myasthenia gravis are all conditions that may be exacerbated with anticholinergic use.

ELECTROCONVULSIVE THERAPY (ECT)

Mechanism of Action
- ECT triggers seizures by applying pulses of current to the scalp.
- The mechanism of action on symptoms of depression, mania, and psychosis is not fully understood.

Indications
- **Major depressive disorder**
- **Manic episodes**
- **Schizophrenia**
- ECT may be the fastest and most effective therapy for major depression.
- It is generally not used until *after* depressed patients **fail medication trials,** or are **acutely suicidal, homicidal,** or **psychotic.**
- Approximately 70 percent of patients with MDD that fail medication trials will respond to ECT.

Side Effects
- Side effects include **headache, confusion,** and **transient memory loss.**
- Memory loss usually resolves within 6 months.

Dosage and Administration
- Treatments are usually given 2 to 3 times per week for 6 to 12 treatments until the maximum therapeutic response is achieved.

Precautions
- There are no *absolute* contraindications to ECT.
- **Increased intracranial pressure, cerebrovascular disease, space-occupying lesions,** and **hypertension** are all *relative* contraindications.

THYROID HORMONE

Mechanism of Action
- The use of thyroid hormone is based on findings that hypothalamic/pituitary/adrenal axis functioning is disturbed in *depressed* patients.
- The precise mechanism of action on symptoms of depression is unclear.
- Liothyronine (Cytomel) is an isomer of triiodothyronine (T_3).
- Levothyroxine (Synthroid) is an isomer of thyroxine (T_4).

Indications
- Adjunctive treatment of **depression**
- Adjunctive treatment of **rapid-cycling bipolar disorder**
- **Lithium-induced hypothyroidism**

Side Effects
- Adverse effects of thyroid hormone are consistent with classic features of hyperthyroidism: diarrhea, weight loss, palpitations, nervousness, sweating, tachycardia, hypertension, tremors, and insomnia.

Thyroid Hormone (continued)

Pharmacokinetics

- The half-life of liothyronine is 1 to 2 days.
- The half-life of levothyroxine is 6 to 7 days.

Dosage and Administration

- An adequate trial should last 1 to 2 weeks.

Precautions

- Thyroid hormone is contraindicated with cardiac disease, hypertension, and hyperthyroidism.

Index

Index

Index